HEALTH SPACES

A PICTORIAL REVIEW

VOLUME 1

HEALTH SPACES

VOLUME 1

A PICTORIAL REVIEW

ISBN 1 8647003-5-1
© 2000
The Images Publishing Group Pty Ltd
Melbourne, Australia 2000
Printed by Leefung-Asco Printers

Contents

A Pictorial Review

Aged Care hospices

Alternative medicine suites

Consulting rooms

Emergency rooms

Intensive Care unit's

Laboratories

Operating theatres

Physiotherapy rooms

Recovery rooms

Rehabilitation/Detoxification centres

Waiting areas

Wards

X-ray/Scanning facilities

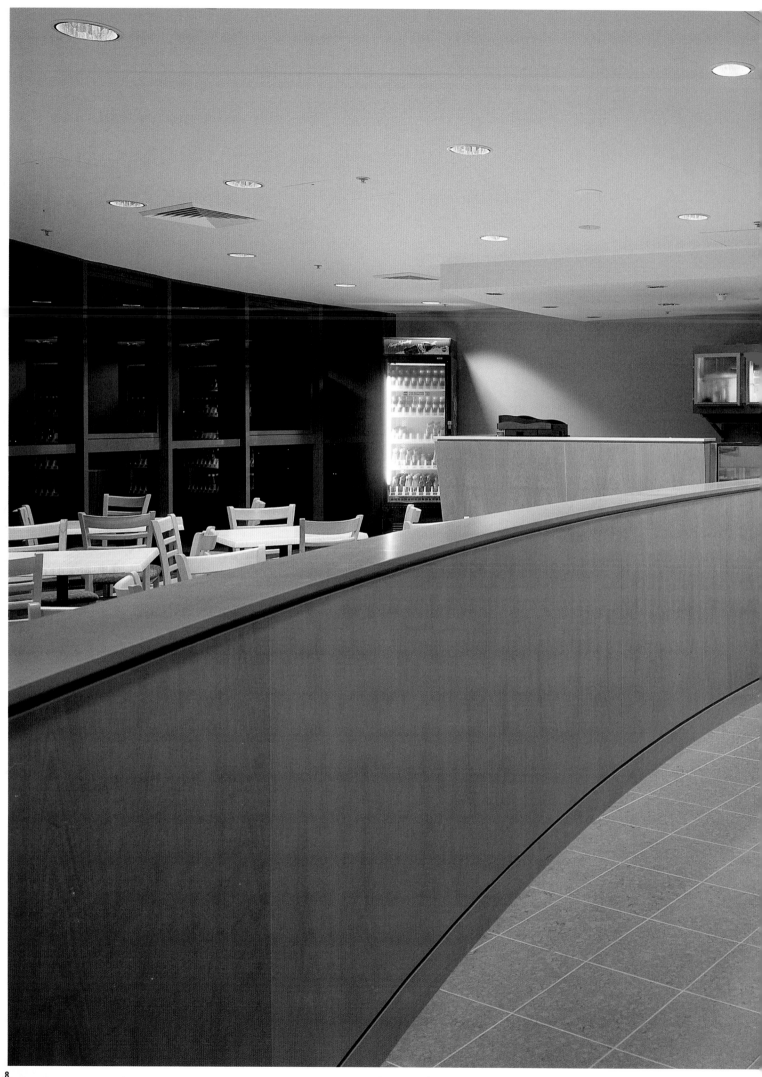

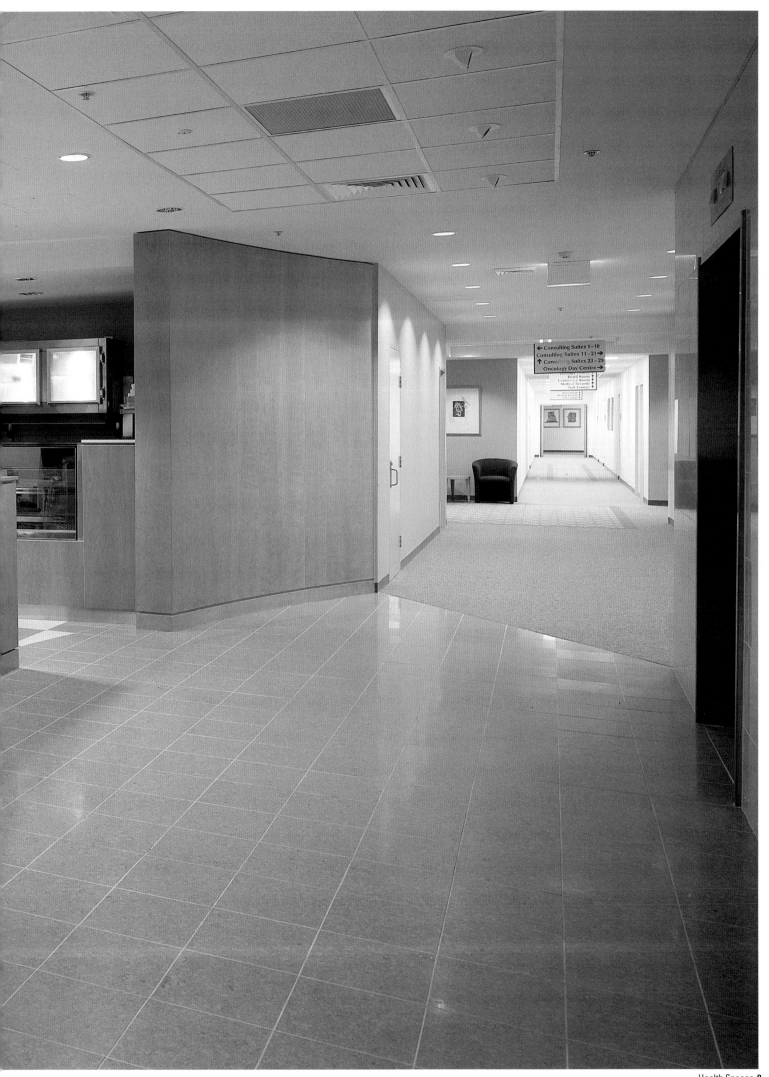

Consulting Suites 1–10 ←
Consulting Suites 11–21 →
↑ Consulting Suites 23–29
Oncology Day Centre →

Board Room ↑
Conference Room ↑
Medical Records ↑
Staff Lounge ↑

**Prince of Wales Hospital
Randwick, NSW, Australia**
Woods Bagot

Previous pages:
    Lift lobby and coffee shop to left
2   Lift lobby
3&4 Cardiology consulting suite
5   Obstetric ward
6   Admissions lift lobby
7   Waiting area
Photo credit: Bart Maiorana

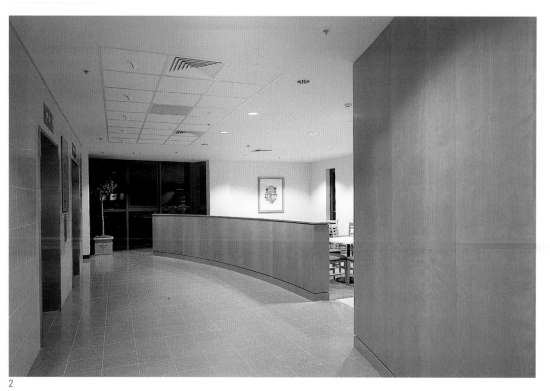

2

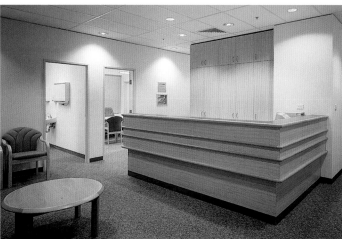

3

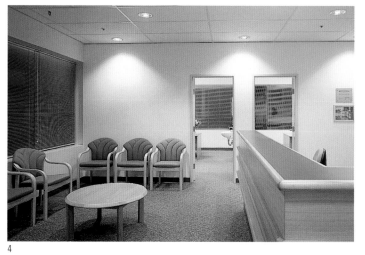

4

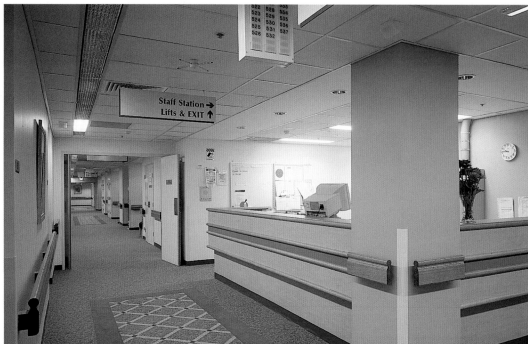

5

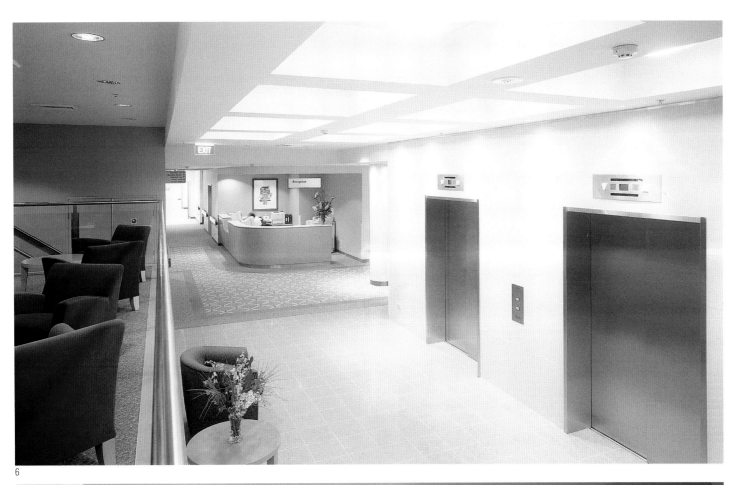

6

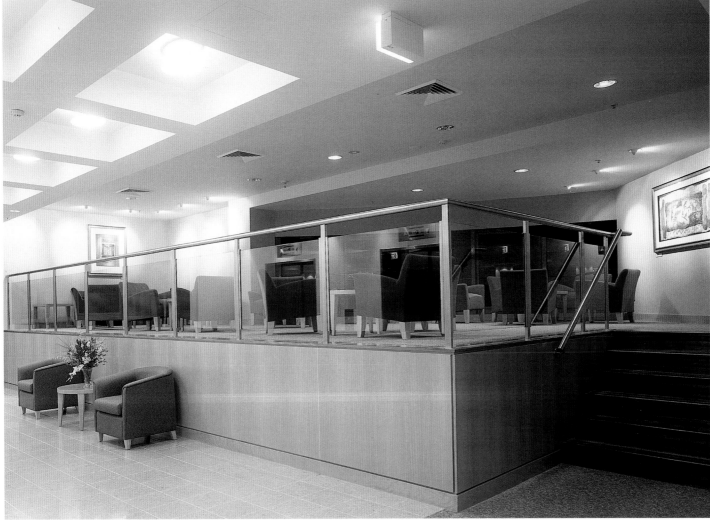

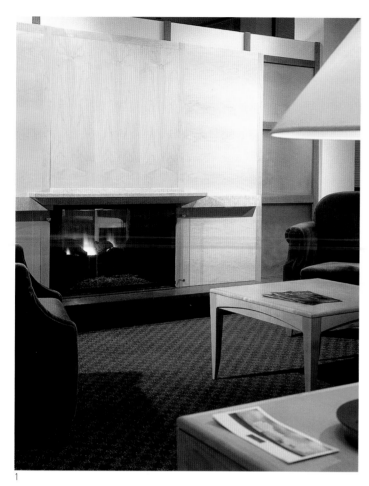

1

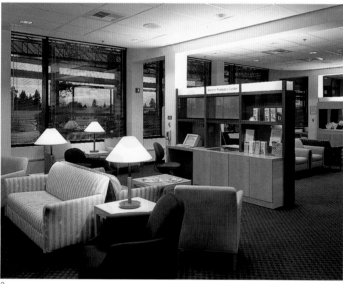

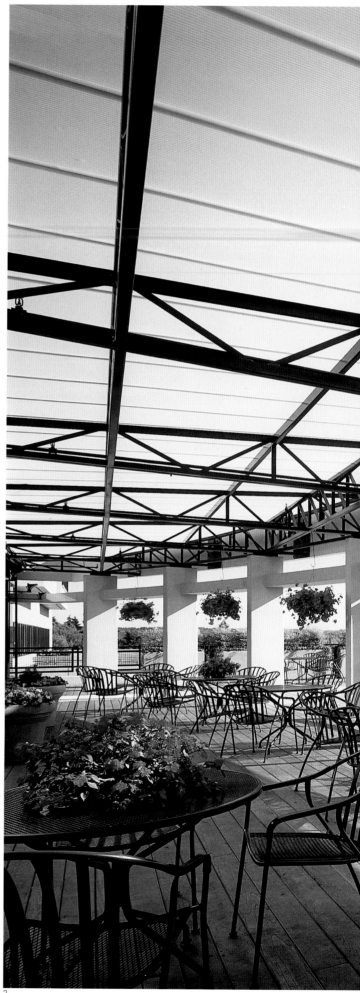

2

Harrison Memorial Hospital
Bremerton, Washington, USA
NBBJ

1   Quiet waiting area and Health Education Center
2   Waiting area
3   Deck and rooftop garden
Photo credits: Paul Warchol (1&2); Assassi Productions (3)

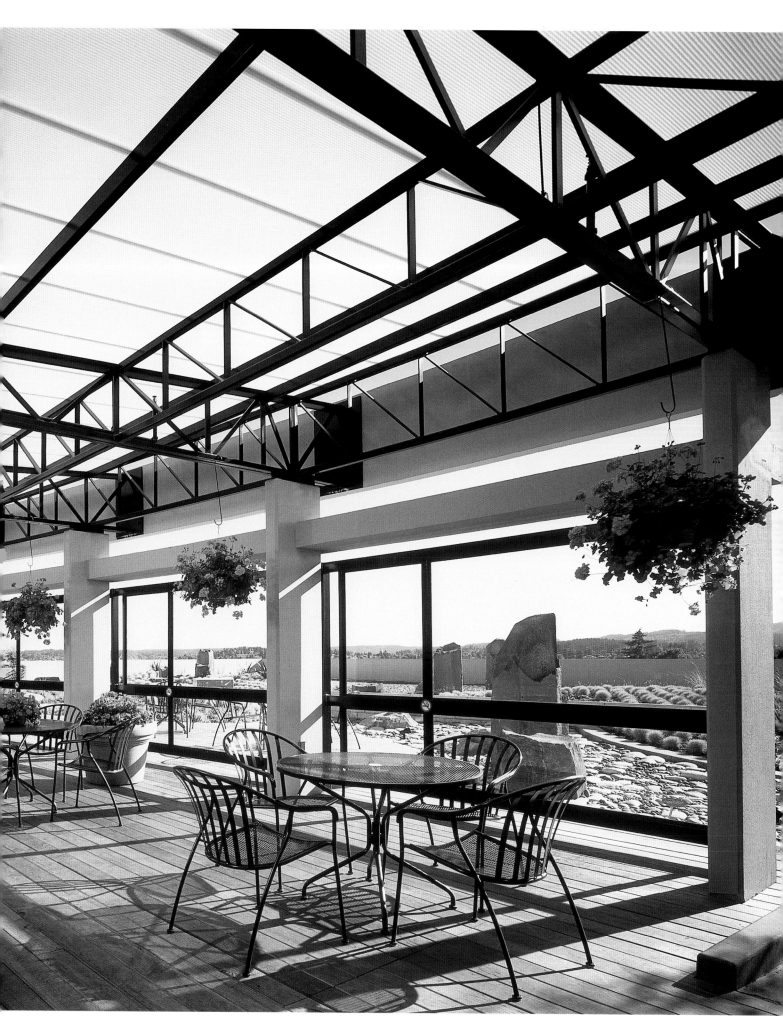

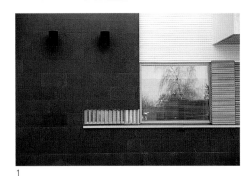

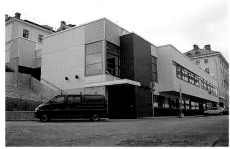

1

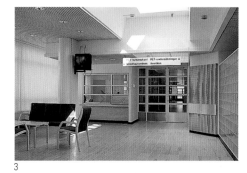

2

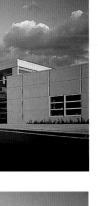

3

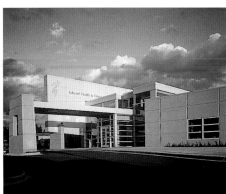

4

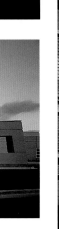

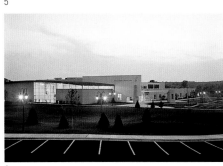

5

6

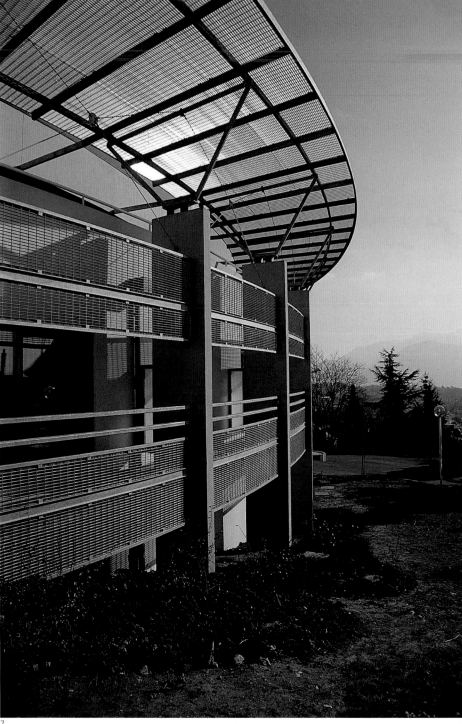

7

National PET Center
Helsinki, Finland
Paatela & Paatela Architects

1   Detail of north elevation
2   View from northeast
3   Entrance lobby
Photo credit: courtesy of Paatela & Paatela Architects

Edward Health and Fitness Centre at Seven Bridges
Woodridge, Illinois, USA
Phillips Swager Associates

4&5   Main entry
6   Exterior view of main building
Photo credit: Barry Rustin Photography

Voiron-Grenoble Hospital
Grenoble, France
BDP Groupe 6

7   Exterior view of extension of general hospital
Photo credit: courtesy of BDP Groupe 6

Avista Hospital
Louisville, Colorado, USA
Davis Partnership P.C., Architects

8   Exterior of hospital at dusk
Photo credit: courtesy of Davis Partnership P.C., Architects

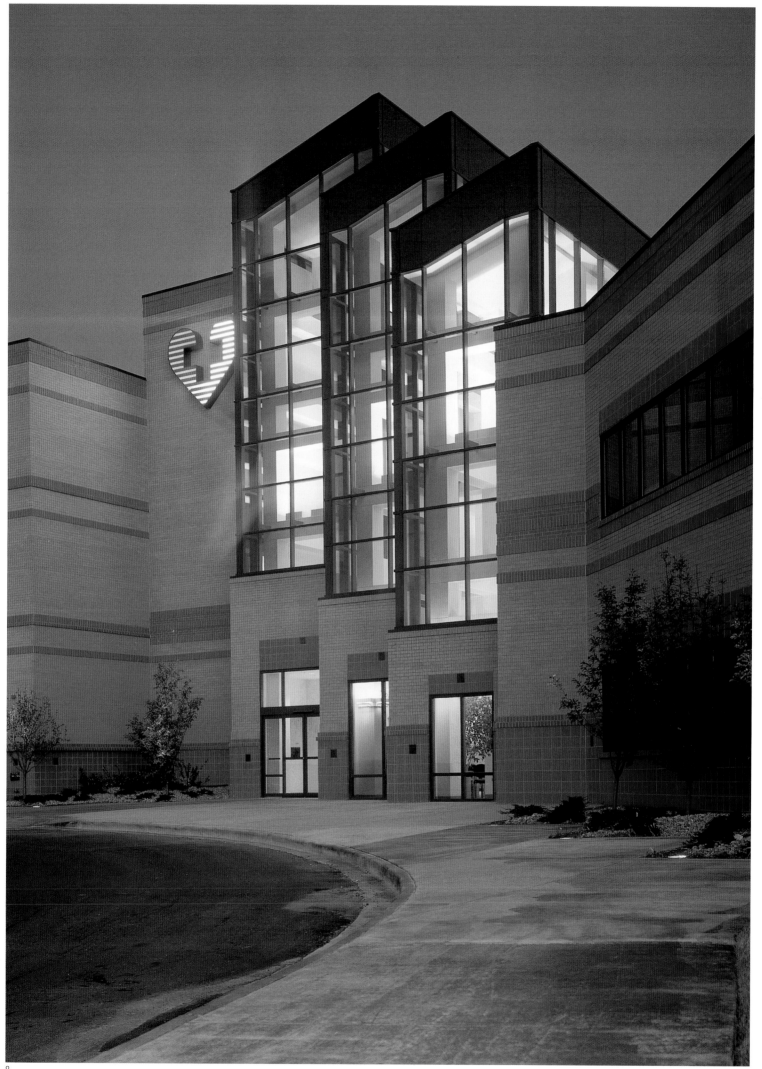

Doernbecher Children's Hospital, Oregon Health Sciences University
Portland, Oregon, USA
Zimmer Gunsul Frasca Partnership in association with Anshen + Allen

1 Main circulation corridors are located along east elevation
2 Hospital spans a canyon, connecting north and south of OHSU campus
3 Main entrance
Photo credit: Timothy Hursley (1&2); Eckert & Eckert Photographic (3)

St. Michael's Hospital
Stevens Point, Wisconsin, USA
Flad & Associates

4 Pedestrian walkway preserves views, access to historic church
Photo credit: Christopher Barrett

University of Wisconsin Hospital & Clinics–West Clinic
Madison, Wisconsin, USA
Flad & Associates

5 Design features natural light for aesthetics and energy efficiency
Photo credit: Christopher Barrett

Anne Arundel Medical Center, Rebecca M. Clatanoff Women's Hospital
Maryland, USA
RTKL Associates Inc.

6 Main entrance forecourt
7 Main atrium lobby
Photo credit: Max MacKenzie

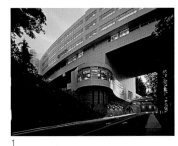
1

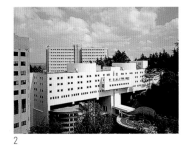
2

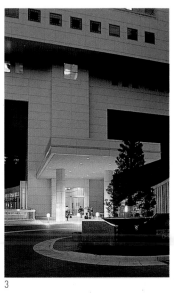
3

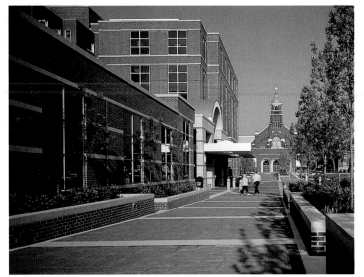
4

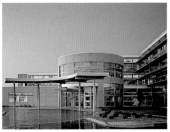
5

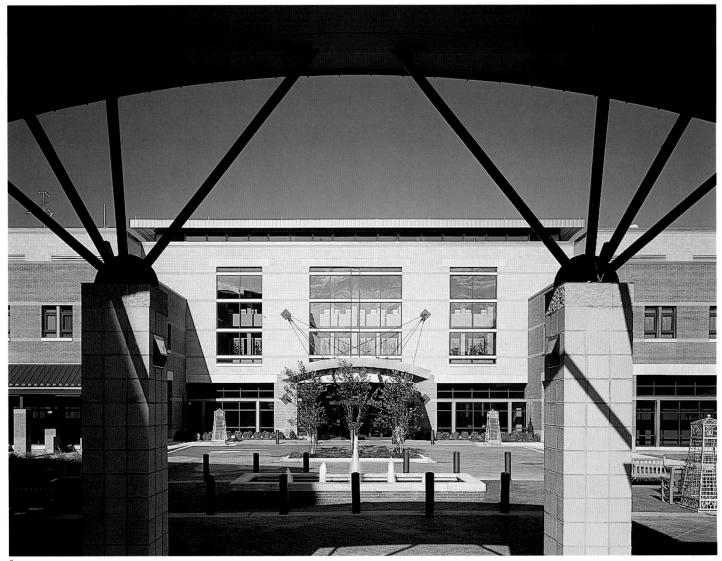

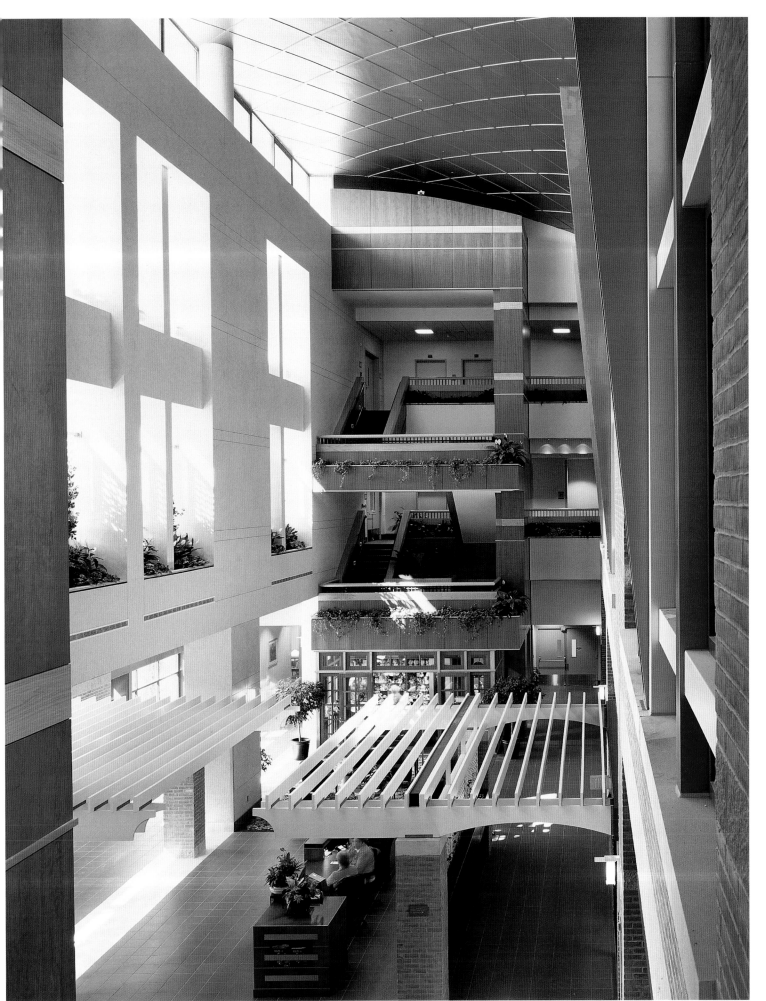

Prudential Health Care System HMO
Lithonia, Georgia, USA
Quantrell Mullins & Associates Inc.
1   Consulting room
2   Corridor to examining rooms
Photo credit: Brian Robbins

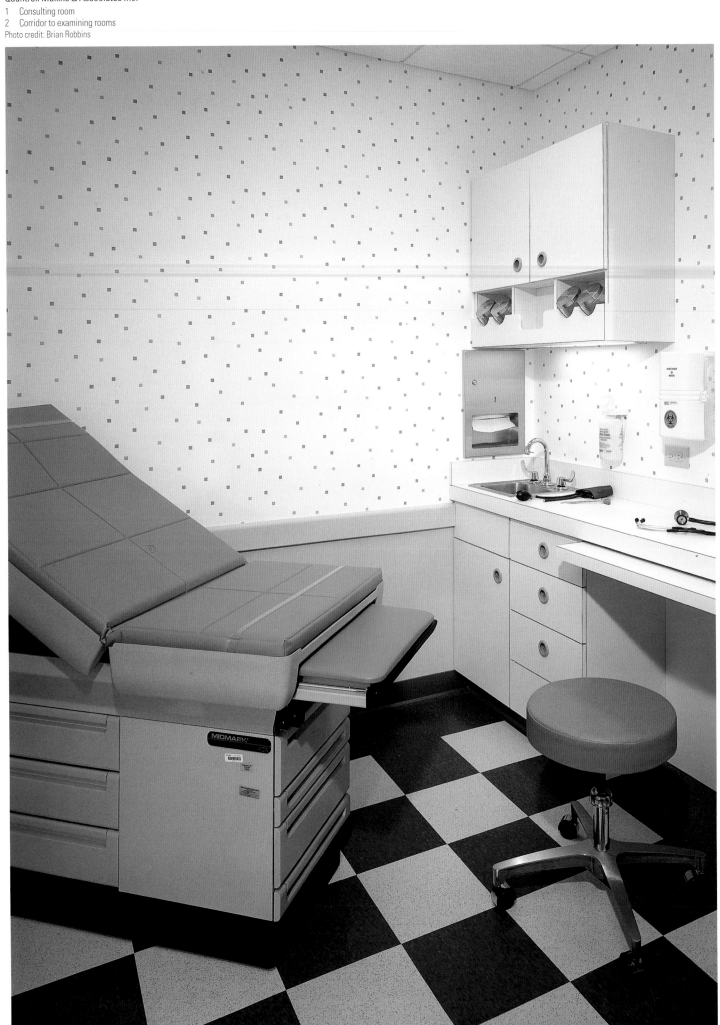

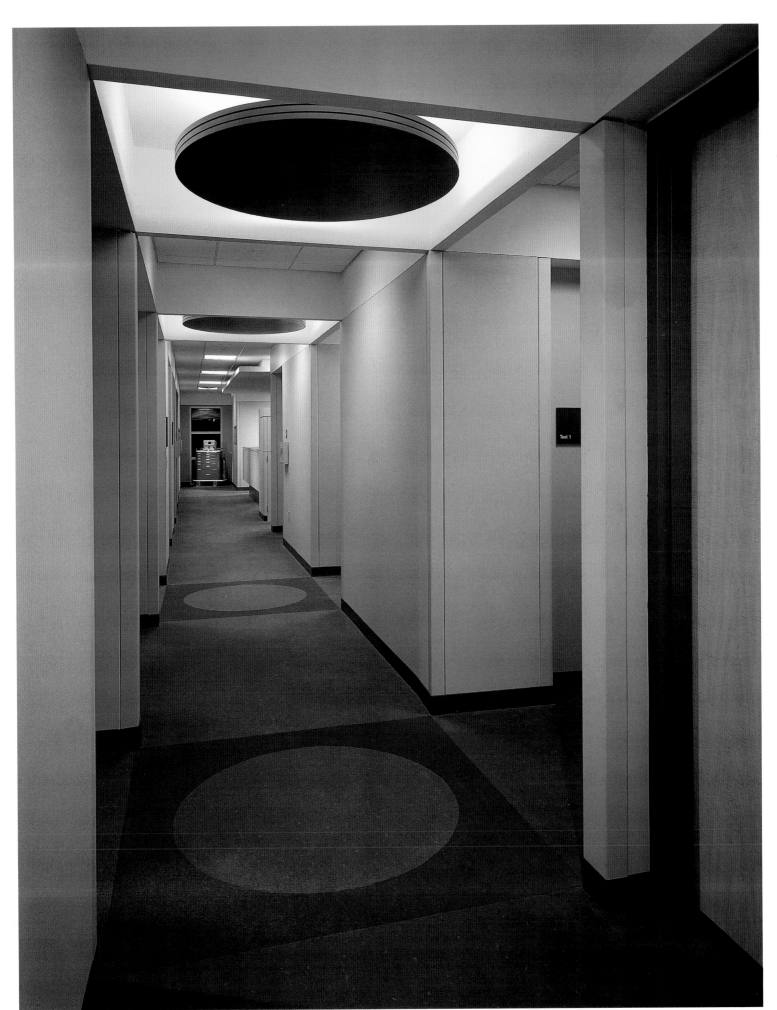

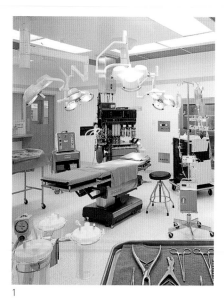

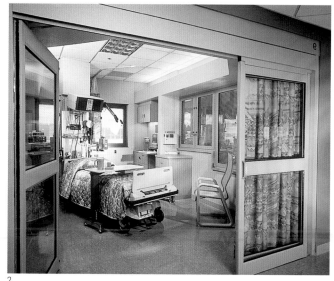

1

2

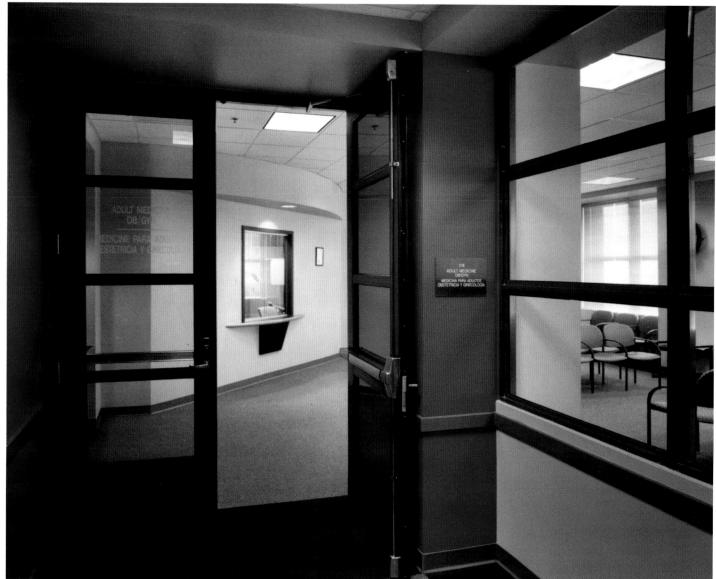

3

Hinsdale Hospital
Hinsdale, Illinois, USA
Loebl Schlossman & Hackl

1   Operating room–Orthopedic Department
Photo credit: Mark Ballogg, Steinkamp/Ballogg
Photography

St. John's Regional Medical Center
Oxnard, California, USA
HKS Inc.

2   Intensive Care Unit
Photo credit: Peter Malinowski

Community Health Services
Connecticut, USA
Du Bose Associates, Inc., Architects

3   Individual specialties are treated as private
physician offices
Photo credit: Robert Benson Photography

Loma Linda University Medical Center
Loma Linda, California, USA
NBBJ

4   Intensive Care Unit at children's
hospital
Photo credit: Michael Shopenn

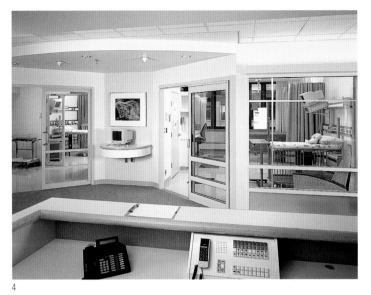

4

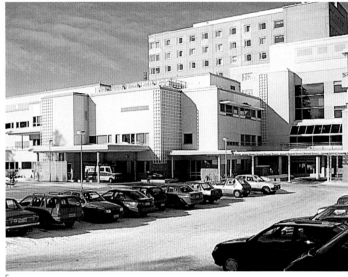

5

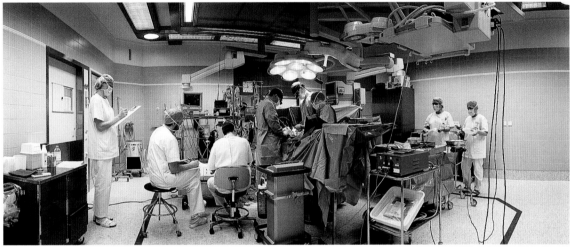

6

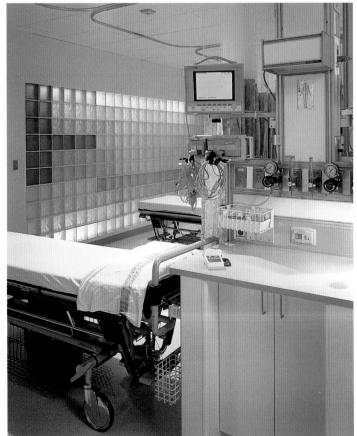

7

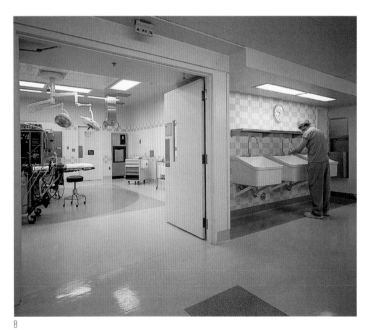

8

Vaasa Central Hospital
Vaasa, Finland
Paatela & Paatela Architects

5   Entrance of Emergency Department
    and Intensive Care Unit
6   Open-heart surgery operating theatre
Photo credit: Risto Laine (5); Unto Heinonen (6)

Swedish Medical Center
Seattle, Washington, USA
NBBJ

7   Ambulatory Care Center's Intensive Care Unit
8   Ambulatory Care Center's operating room
    and scrub area
Photo credit: Assassi Productions

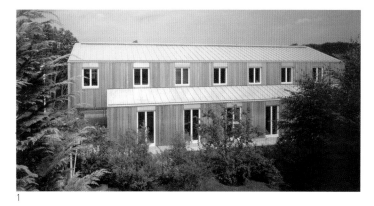

1

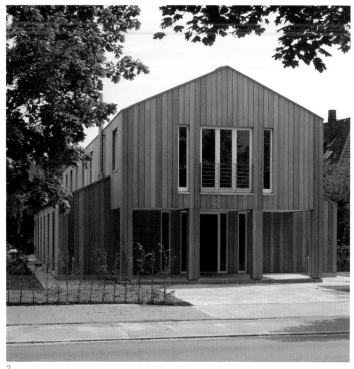

2

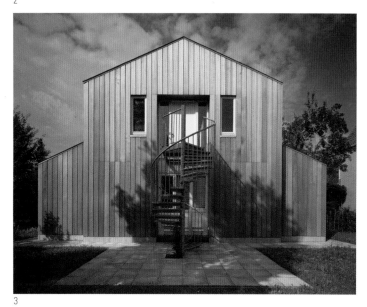

3

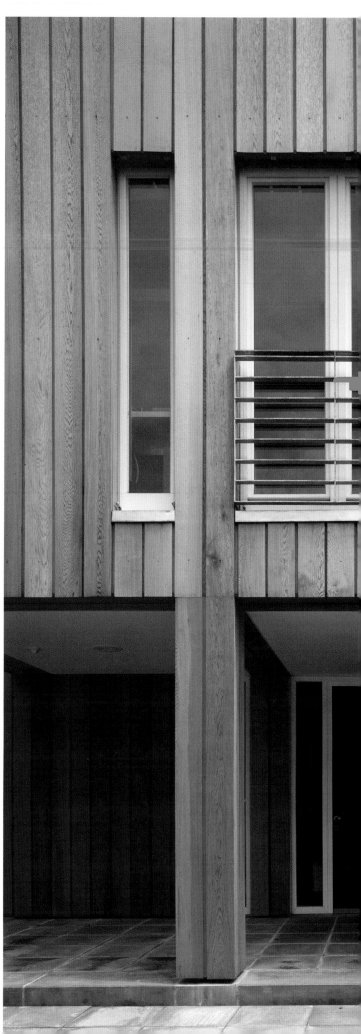

Dr. Med. Manke Consulting Office
Uelzen, Germany

gmp–von Gerkan Marg & Partner

1   Façade in red cedar and sheet-zinc roof
    cladding
2   Strict composition is based on building's
    cross-section which resembles a
    basilica

3   Rear elevation with spiral stair leading
    to small apartment
4   Front elevation
5   Central corridor for patients
6   System of sliding doors offers doctor
    quick access and surveillance over four
    surgeries

Photo credit: Klaus Frahm

4

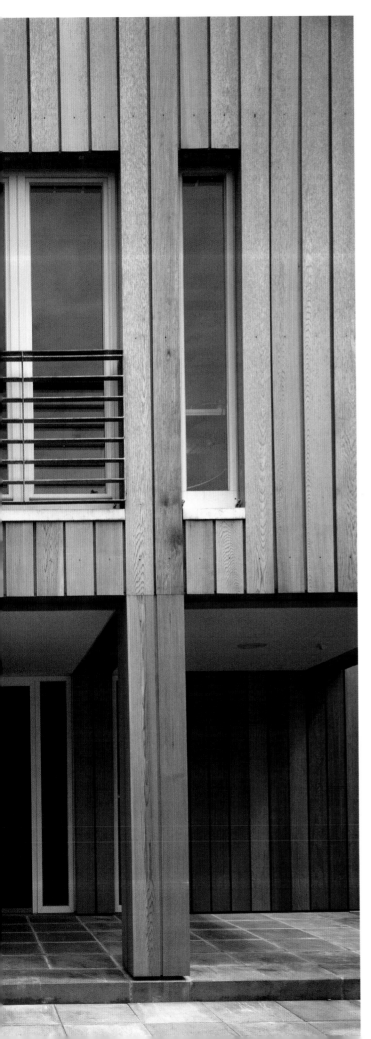

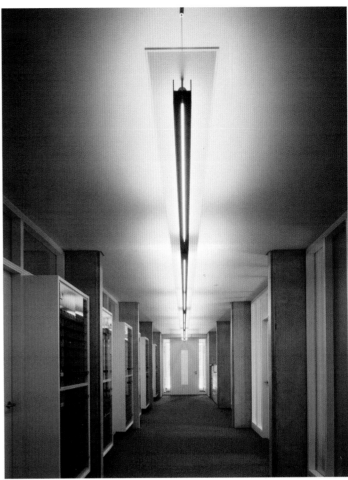

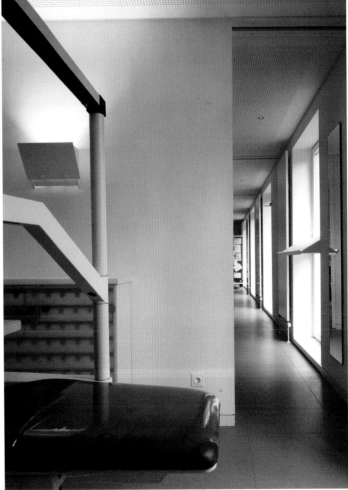

5

6

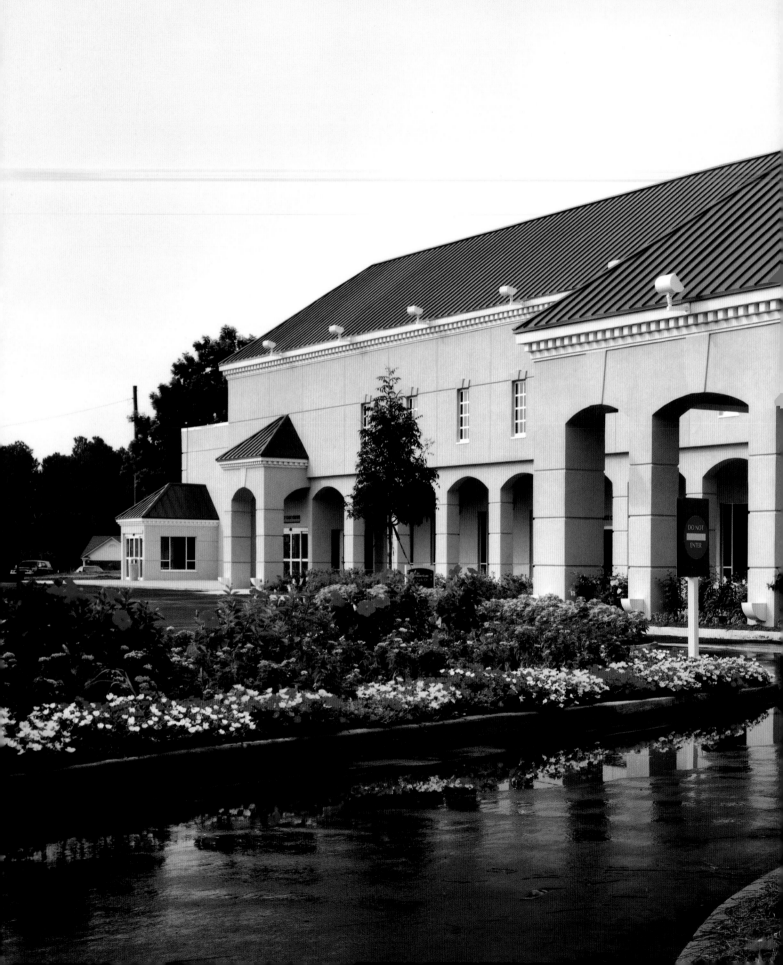

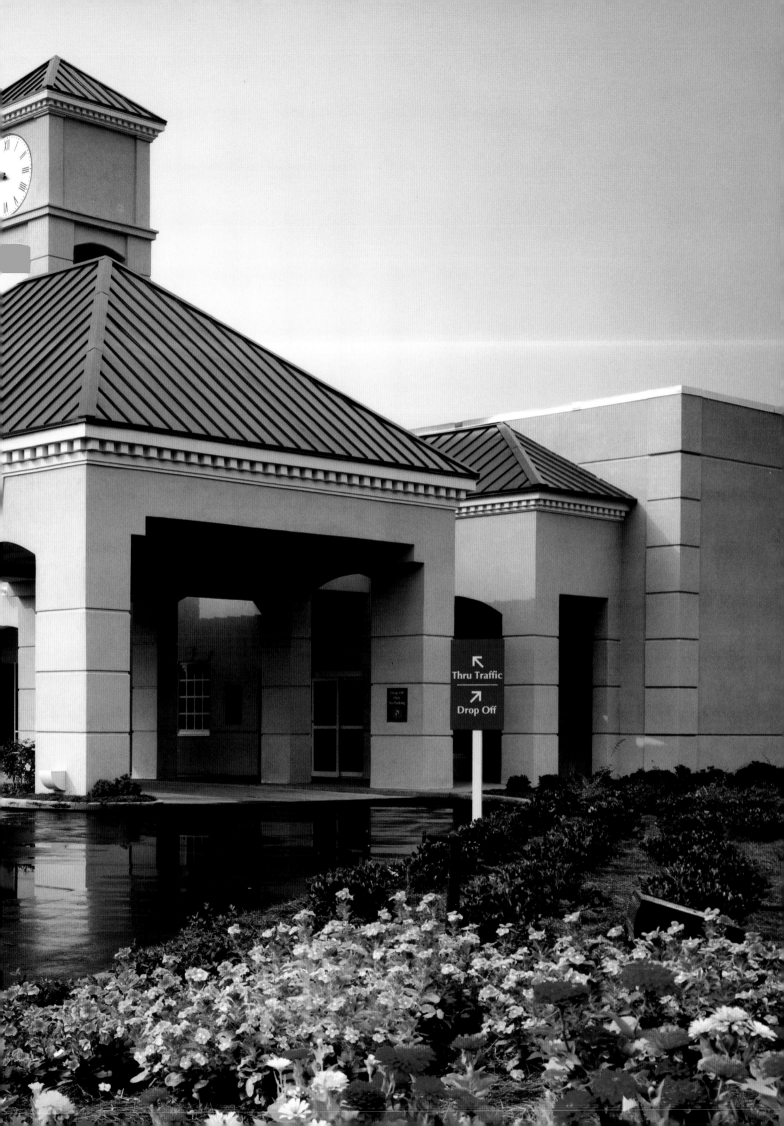

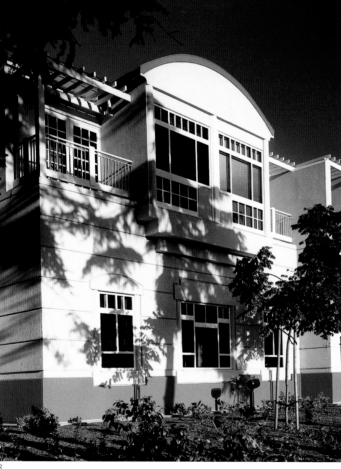

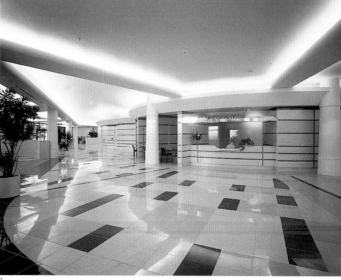

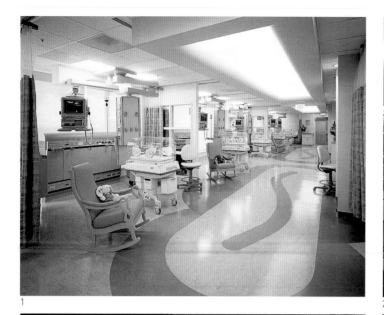

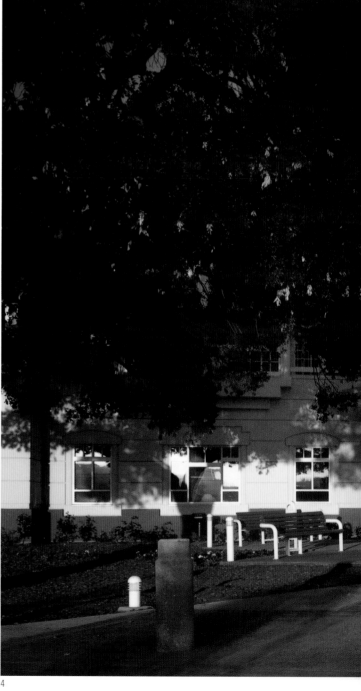

Phoebe Northwest, Phoebe Putney Memorial Hospital
Albany, Georgia, USA
TRO/The Ritchie Organization

Previous pages:
    Dramatic renovation of abandoned supermarket, exterior view
Photo credit: George Cott

Utah Valley Regional Medical Center's Women's and Children's Addition
Provo, Utah, USA
HKS Inc. in association with Design West

1   Neonatal
2   Public space
Photo credit: Ed LaCasse

Sutter Santa Cruz Maternity and Surgical Center
Santa Cruz, California, USA
Kaplan McLaughlin Diaz in association with Silva Strong Architects

3   Existing grove of redwoods and heritage oaks cast bold shadows on front facade
4&5   Entrance rotunda serves to unite building's two wings
6   Dining and conference room faces rear yard
Photo credit: Erich Anset Koyama

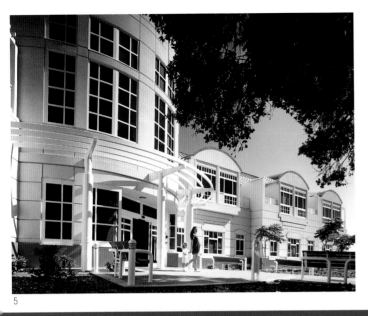

5

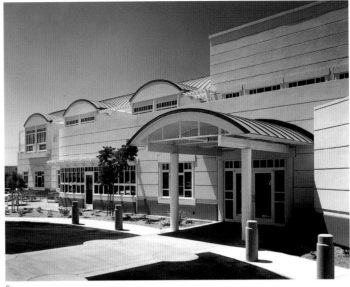

6

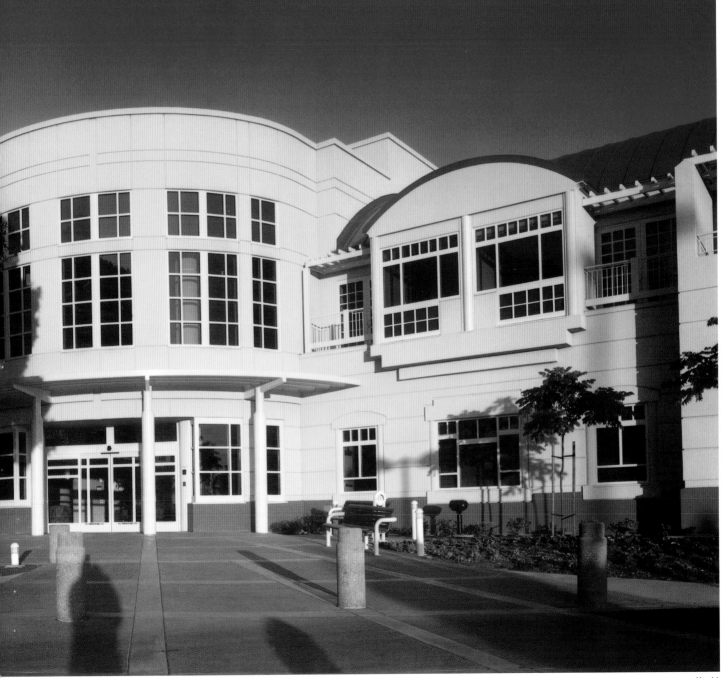

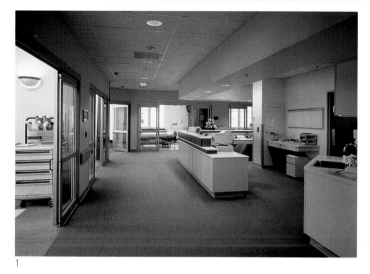

1

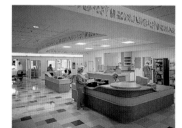

2

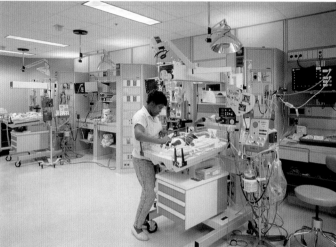

3

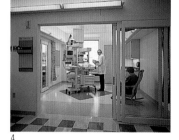

4

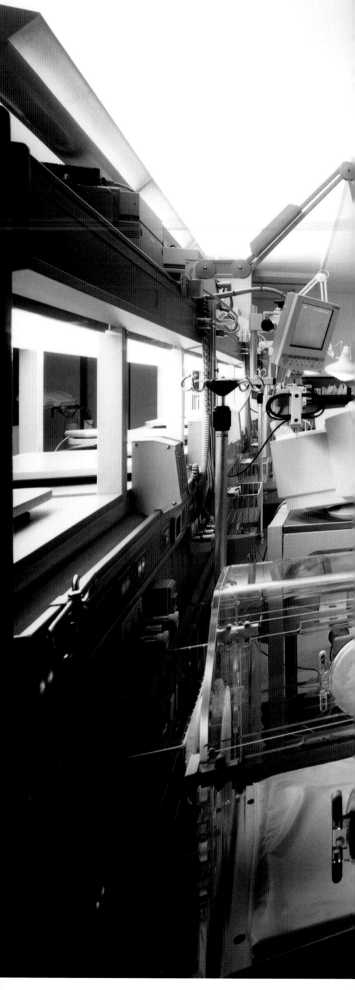

St. Mary's Hospital
Ozaukee, Mequon, Wisconsin, USA
HKS Inc.
1   Intensive Care Unit
Photo credit: Rick Grumbaum

Children's Medical Center
Dallas, Texas, USA
HKS Inc.
2   Neonatal Intensive Care Unit
Photo credit: Rick Grumbaum

Doernbecher Children's Hospital, Oregon
Health Sciences University
Portland, Oregon, USA
Zimmer Gunsul Frasca Partnership in
association with Anshen + Allen
3   Hand stenciled artwork is incorporated
      throughout hospital including Paediatric
      Intensive Care Unit
4   Paediatric Intensive Care Unit Patient Rooms
Photo credit: Eckert & Eckert Photographic

The New York Hospital
New York, USA
Hellmuth, Obata + Kassabaum, Inc.
5   Neonatal Intensive Care Unit
Photo credit: courtesy of Hellmuth, Obata +
Kassabaum, Inc.

Alexian Brothers Medical Center
Elk Grove Village, Illinois, USA
Loebl Schlossman & Hackl
Following pages:
    MRI Spaces
Photo credit: Val Studio Photography

5

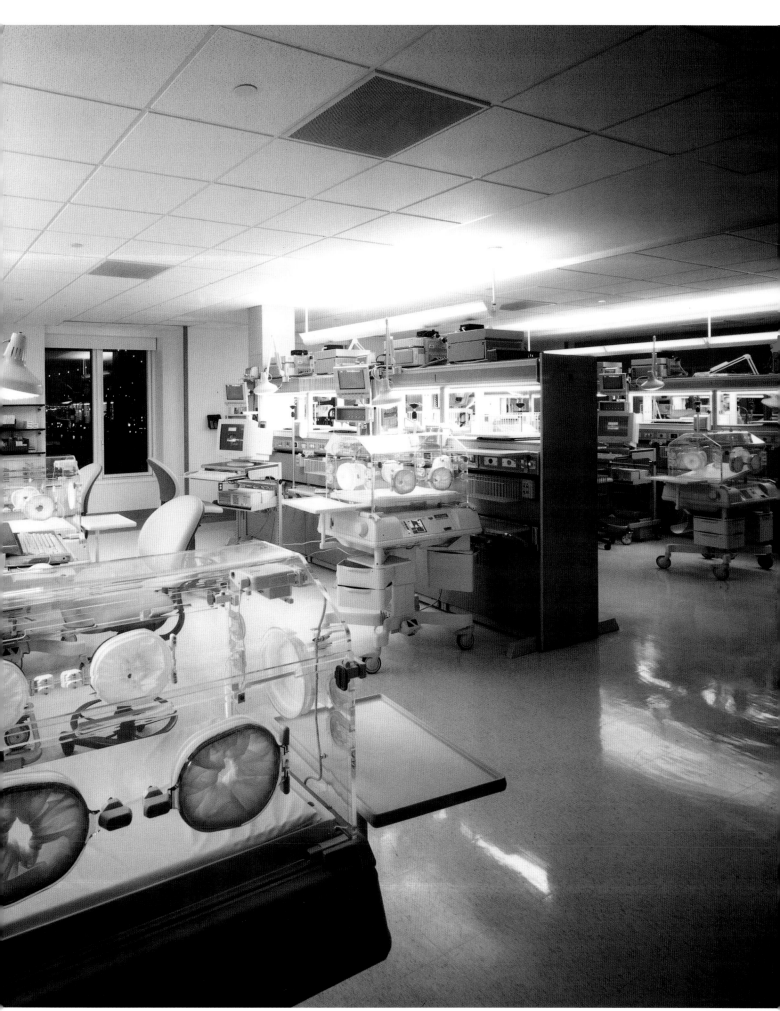

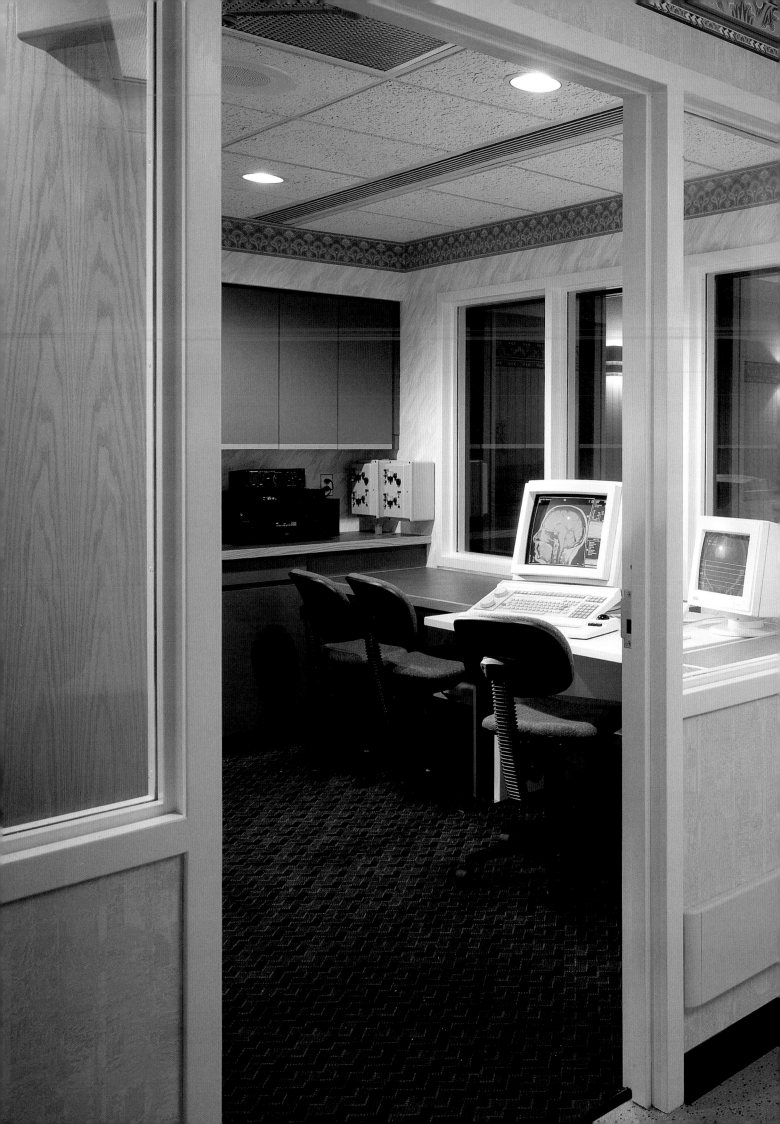

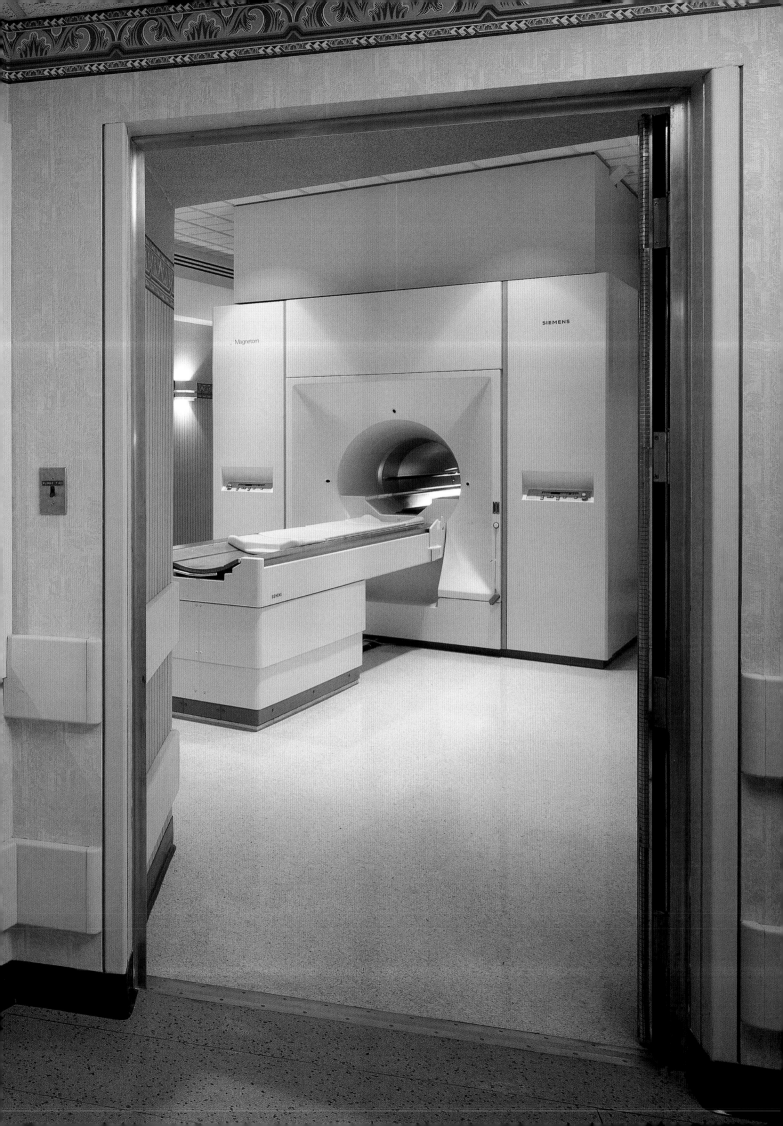

St. Michael's Hospital
Stevens Point, Wisconsin, USA
Flad & Associates
1   Histopathology remains private, yet offers
      view to outdoors
2   Plentiful windows bring light and nature
      across laboratory benches
Photo credit: Christopher Barrett

North Carolina Neuroscience's Hospital,
University of North Carolina
Chapel Hill, North Carolina, USA
HKS Inc.
3&4   Emergency room
Photo credit: Wes Thompson

MD Anderson Cancer Center
Houston, Texas, USA
LAN/HKS Inc. Joint Venture
5   Operating room
Photo credit: Wes Thompson

Maimonides Medical Center,
Sheepshead Bay Primary Care Center
Brooklyn, New York, USA
Lee Harris Pomeroy Associates/Architects
6   'Wave wall' along examination room;
      physician's office corridor
Photo credit: Christopher Lovi

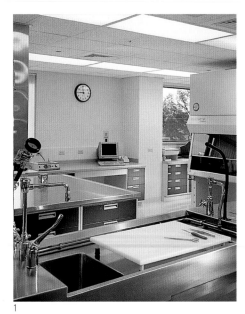
1

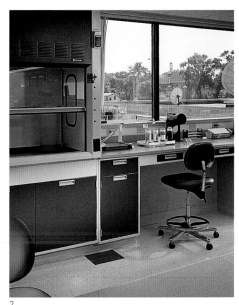
2

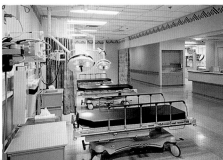
3

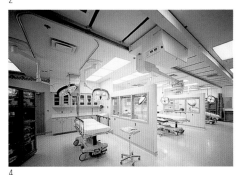
4

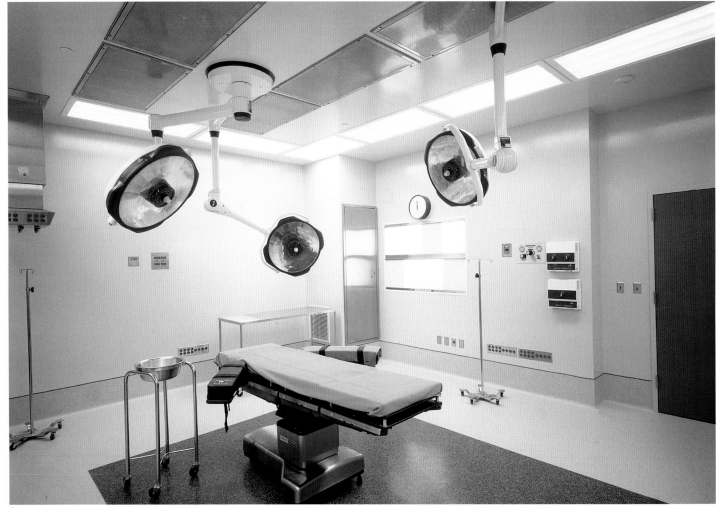

5

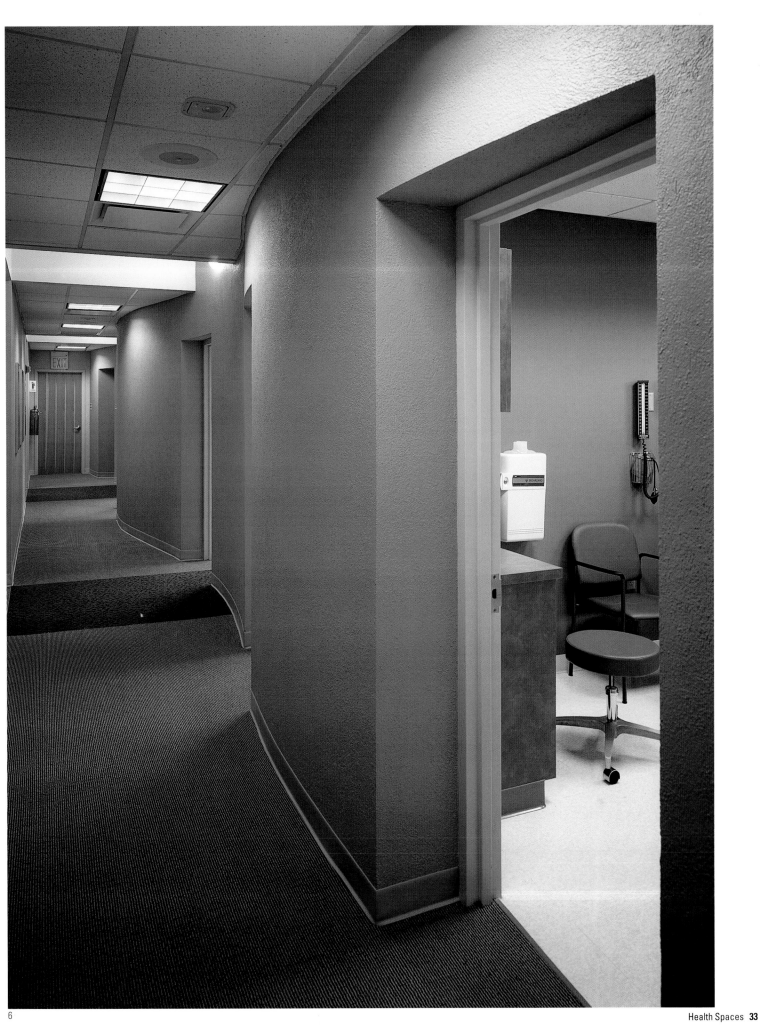

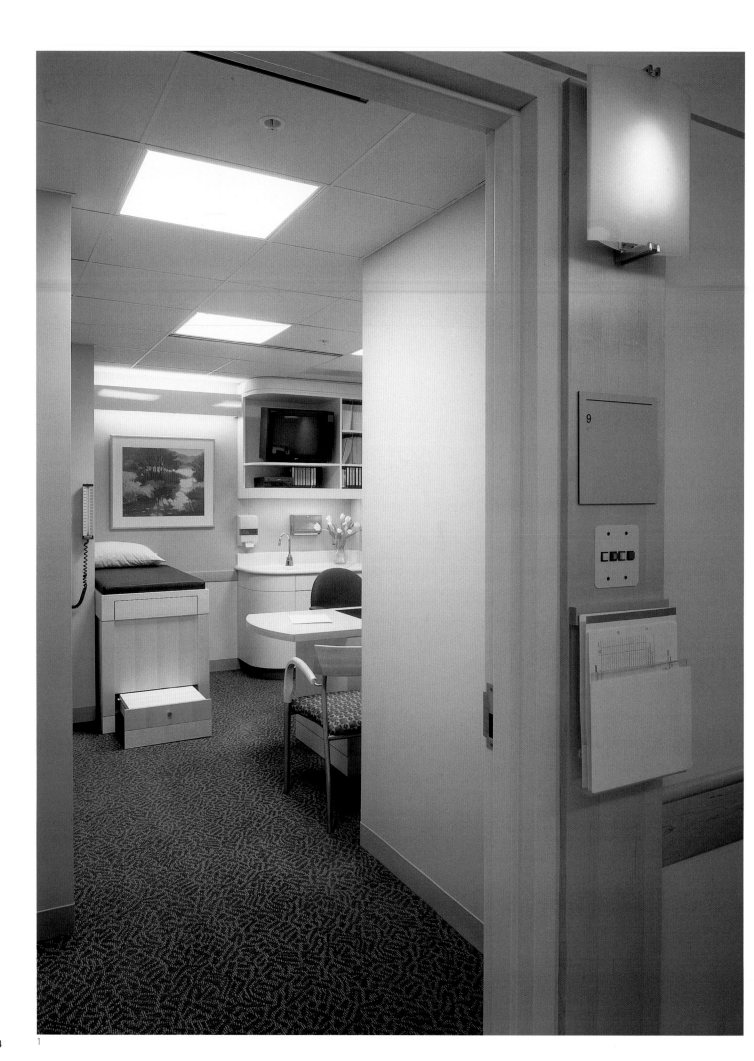

1

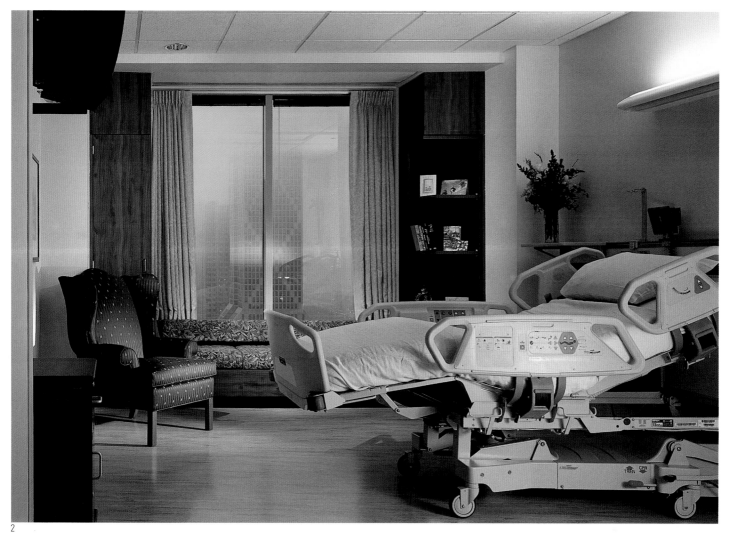

2

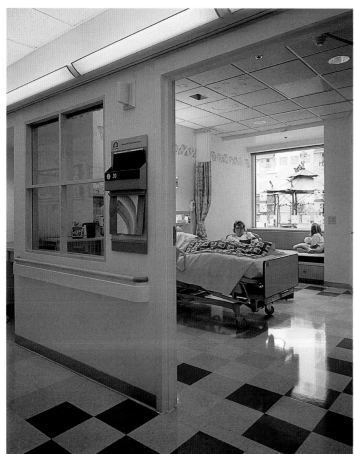

3

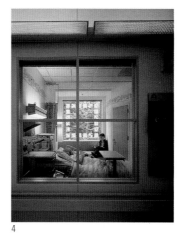

4

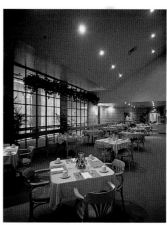

5

**Swedish Medical Center
Seattle, Washington, USA**
NBBJ

1   Ambulatory Care Center consulting room
Photo credit: Steve Keating

**Northwestern Memorial Hospital
Chicago, Illinois, USA**
Hellmuth, Obata + Kassabaum, Inc. in
association with Ellerbe Becket and VOA

2   Home-like atmosphere for patients
Photo credit: Justin Machonochie/Hedrich-
Blessing

**Doernbecher Children's Hospital, Oregon
Health Sciences University
Portland, Oregon, USA**
Zimmer Gunsul Frasca Partnership in
association with Anshen + Allen

3   Patient rooms are organized as
     'neighbourhoods'
4   Each patient room incorporates a window,
     parent bed and artwork
Photo credit: Eckert & Eckert Photographic

**Hearthstone
Sun City, Arizona, USA**
HKS Inc.

5   Dining area
Photo credit: Greg Hursley

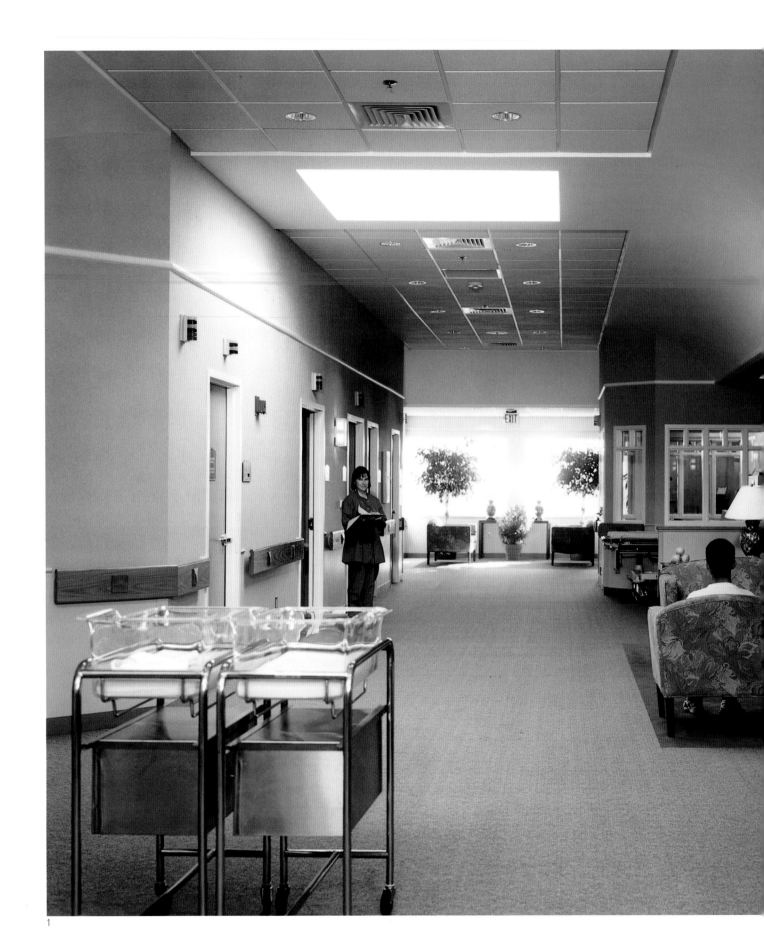

1

Sutter Santa Cruz Maternity and Surgical Center
Santa Cruz, California, USA
Kaplan McLaughlin Diaz in association with Silva
Strong Architects
1   View from second floor through ceiling windows
      to park-like settings
Photo credit: Erich Anset Koyama

Washoe Village Care Center
Reno, Nevada, USA
HKS Inc. in association with Cathexes, Inc.
2   Living suite
3   Social gathering place
Photo credit: Ed LaCasse

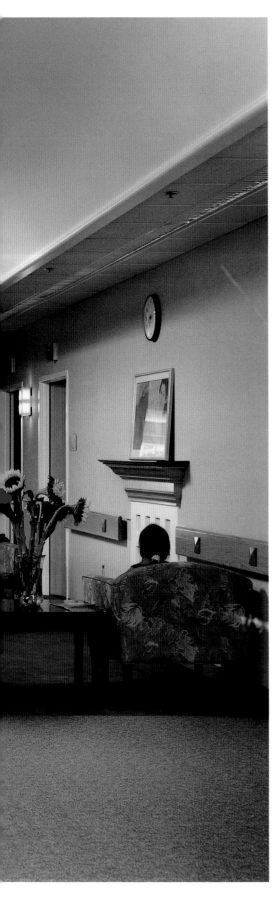

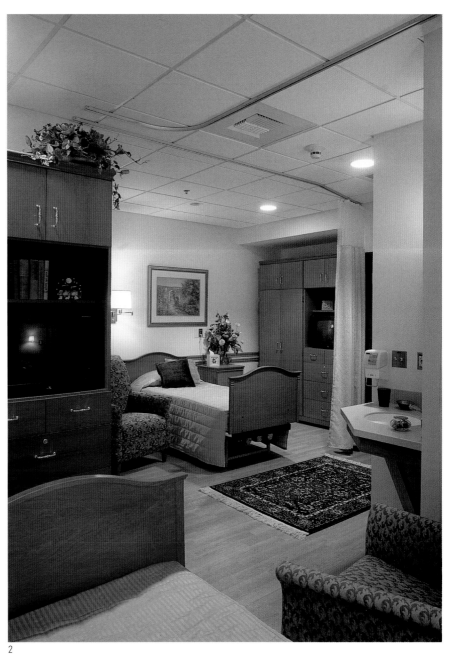

2

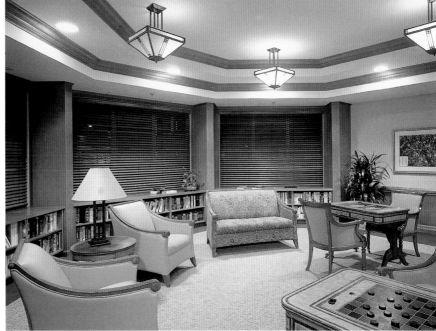

3

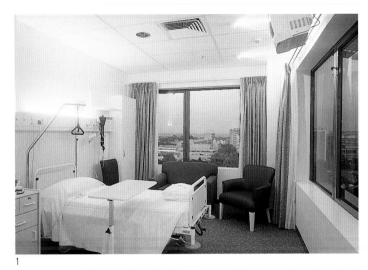

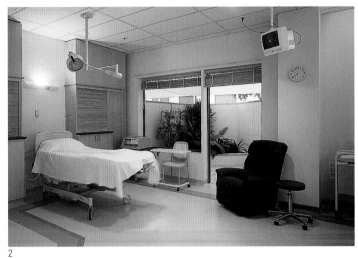

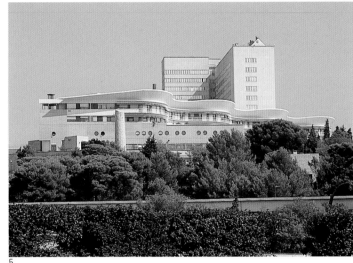

1

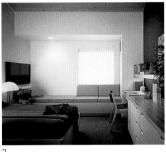

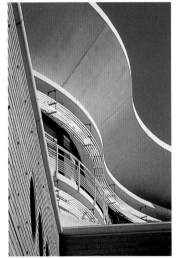

2

3

4   5

Prince of Wales Hospital
Randwick, NSW, Australia
Woods Bagot
   1   Obstetrics ward
   2   Birthing room with private courtyard
Photo credit: Bart Maiorana

Menninger Foundation
Topeka, Kansas, USA
Skidmore, Owings & Merrill LLP
   3   Inpatient psychiatric room
Photo credit: courtesy of Skidmore,
Owings & Merrill LLP

Marseille Hospital
Marseille, France
BDP Groupe 6
   4   Paediatric wing's façade facing
       Mediterranean
   5   Exterior view of paediatric wing and
       teaching hospital
Photo credit: courtesy of BDP Groupe 6

Barry Medical Park
Kansas City, Missouri, USA
WRS Architects Inc.
6&7   Consulting and exam room for Vision
       Correction Center
Photo credit: Mike Sinclair Photography

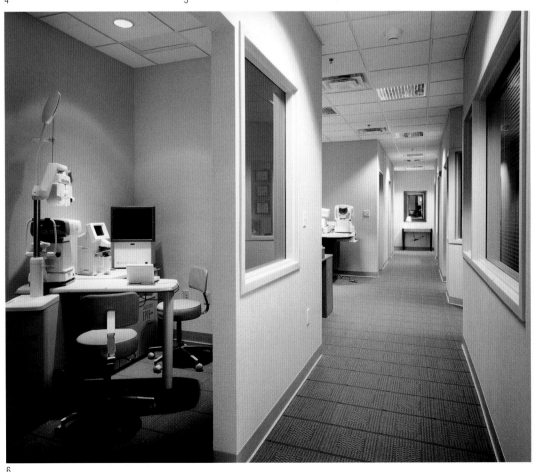

6

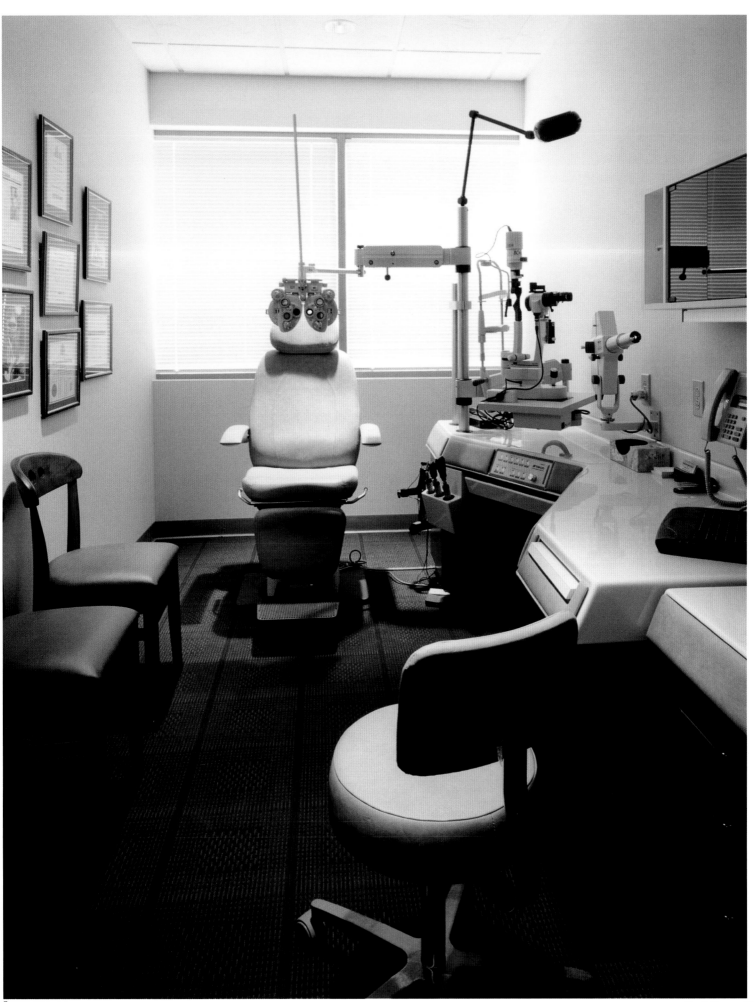

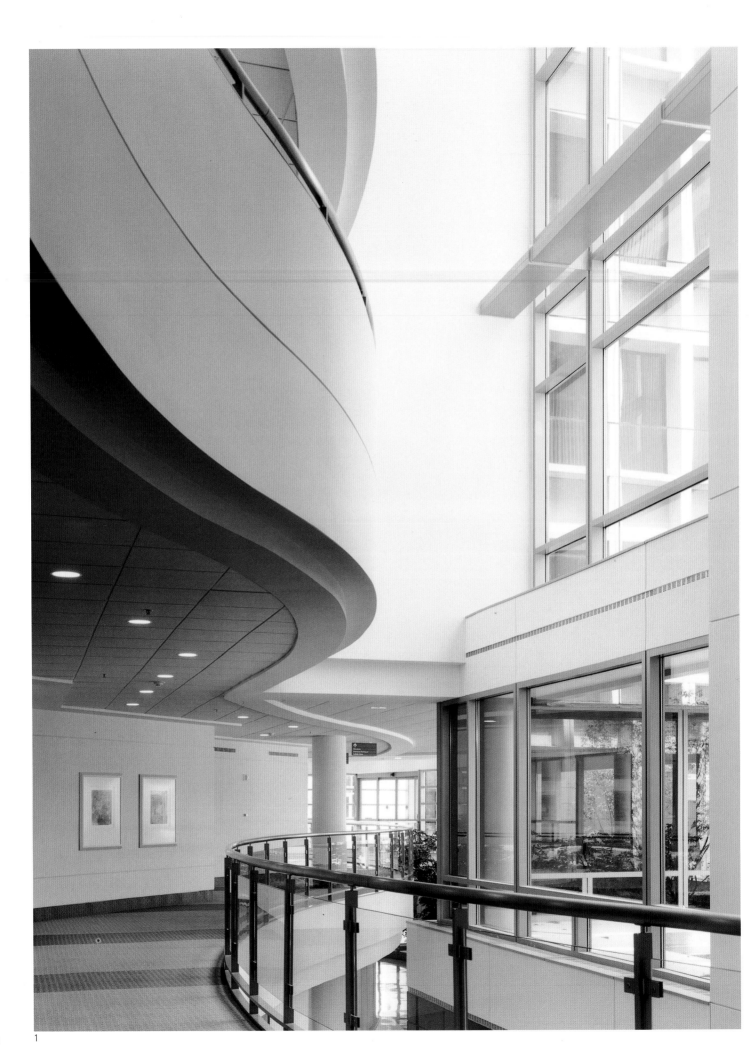

1

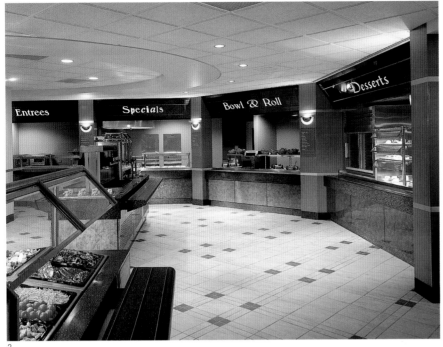

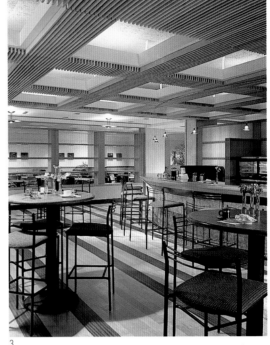

2

3

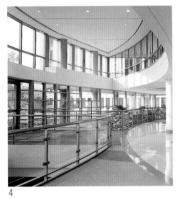

4

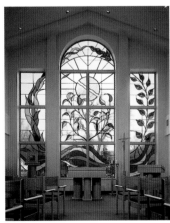

5

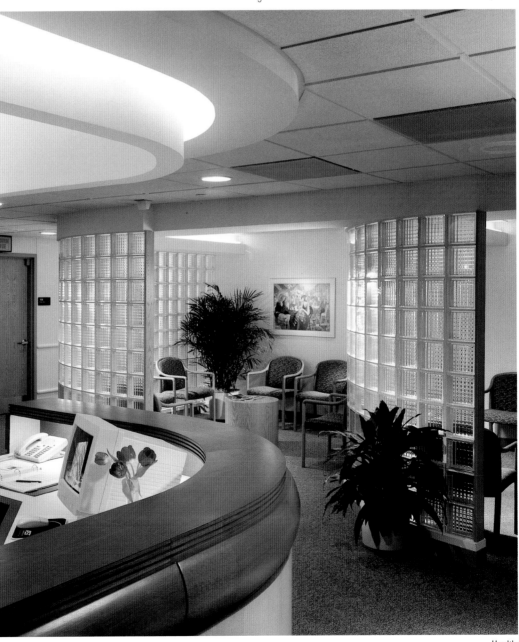

Resurrection Medical Center
Chicago, Illinois, USA
Loebl Schlossman & Hackl

1&4   Professional office building, atrium
        corridor
2   Scatter-system servery
3   Dining facility—cappuccino bar
5   Life Center Chapel

Photo credits: Scott McDonald (3&6); Bruce
VanInwegen (1,2,4–6)

Lutheran General Hospital,
Cancer Care Center
Park Ridge, Illinois, USA
Loebl Schlossman & Hackl

6   Nurses' station/waiting area

Photo credit: Bruce VanInwegen Photography

6

Vaasa Central Hospital
Helsinki, Finland
Paatela & Paatela Architects

1   Patient examination and treatment building
Photo credit: Vaasa Central Hospital

Lowell General Hospital, Cancer Care Center
Lowell, Massachusetts, USA
TRO/The Ritchie Organization

2   Exam rooms are designed for patient comfort and staff efficiency
Photo credit: Edward Jacoby/Jacoby Photography

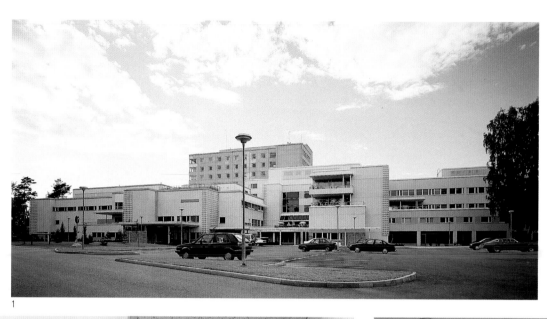

1

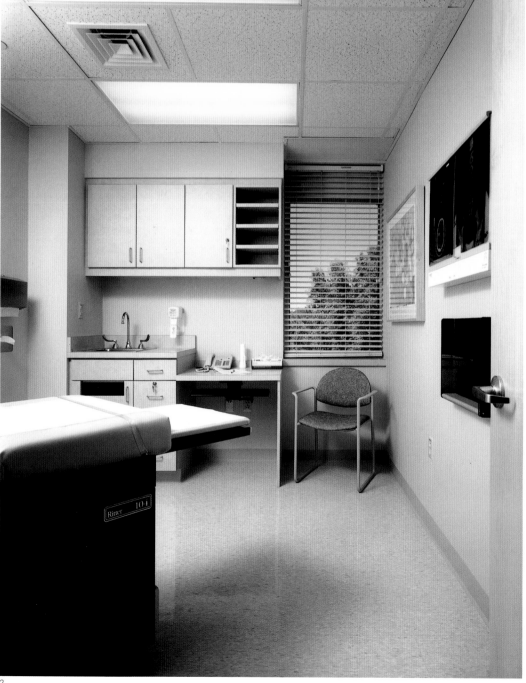

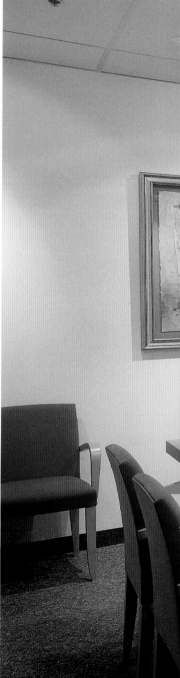

2

3

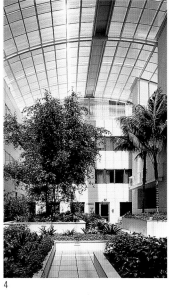

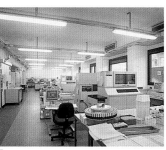

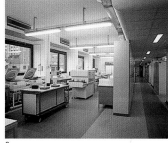

**Prince of Wales Hospital
Randwick, NSW, Australia**
Woods Bagot

3   Executive boardroom
4   Eastern atrium courtyards
Photo credit: Bart Maiorana

**S. Orsola-Malpighi Hospital,
New Centralized Laboratories
Bologna, Italy**
Architetto Belli Patrizia Virginia

5&6   Interior view of second floor space
Photo credit: Simone Ruzzenente

4   5   6

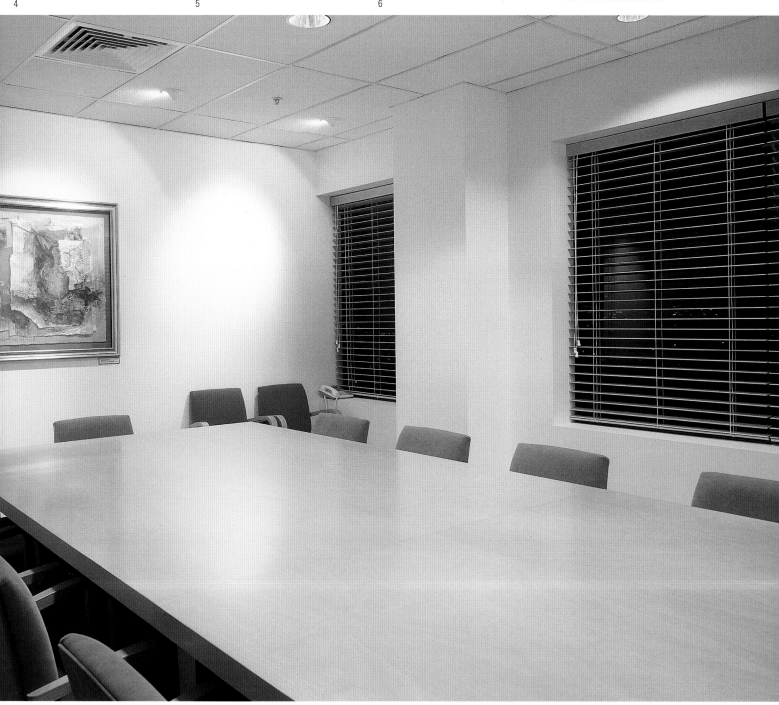

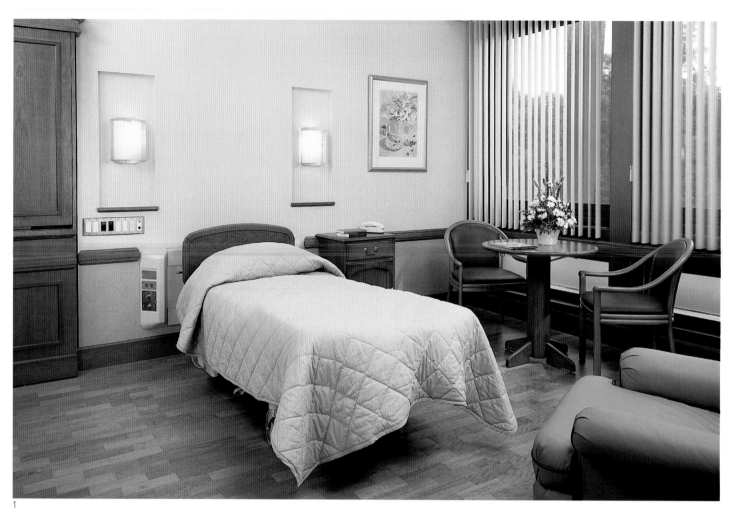

1

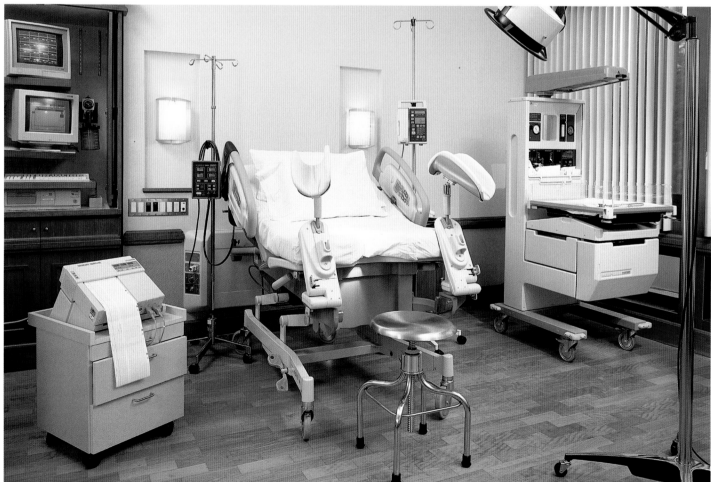

2

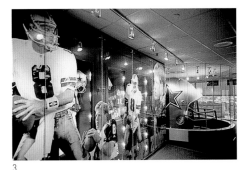

3

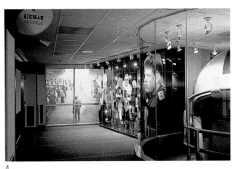

4

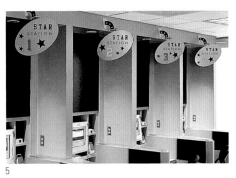

5

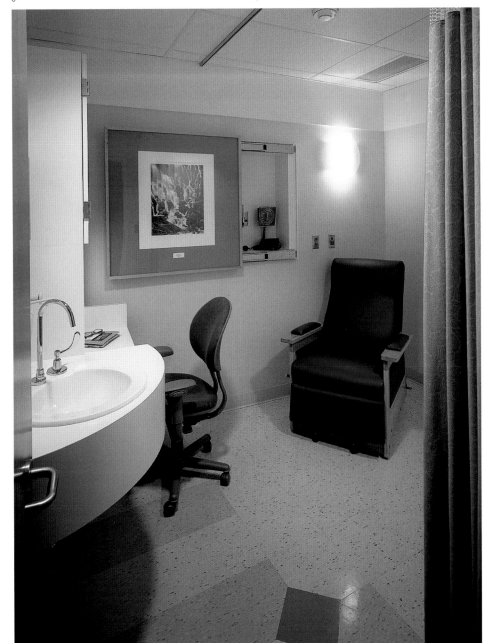

6

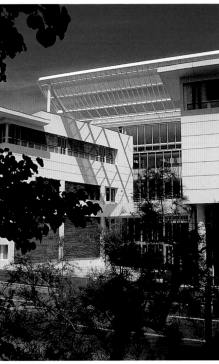

7

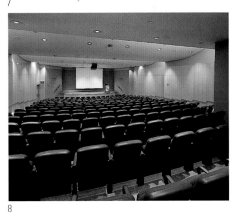

8

Anne Arundel Medical Center, Rebecca M. Clatanoff Women's Hospital Maryland, USA
RTKL Associates Inc.
1 Typical LDRP room
2 Typical LDRP room set-up
Photo credit: Max MacKenzie

Aikman's End Zone, Children's Medical Center of Dallas Dallas, Texas, USA
HKS Inc.
3 Display case, memorabilia wall with eight-foot helmet
4 Corridor leading to Aikman's Avenue
5 'Starbright', interactive computers
Photo credit: Ron St. Angelo

Harrison Memorial Hospital Bremerton, Washington, USA
NBBJ
6 Medical equipment can be hidden in consultation rooms
Photo credit: Steve Keating

Salon de Provence Hospital Salon de Provence, France
BDP Groupe 6
7 Exterior of maternity wing and entrance
Photo credit: courtesy of BDP Groupe 6

Garvan Institute of Medical Research Darlinghurst, NSW, Australia
Ancher Mortlock and Woolley
8 Theatre for conferences
Photo credit: Eric Sierins

Blood Bank and Laboratories Parramatta, NSW, Australia
Ancher Mortlock and Woolley
Following pages:
    Donor room/recovery area
Photo credit: Sierins/Max Dupain & Associates

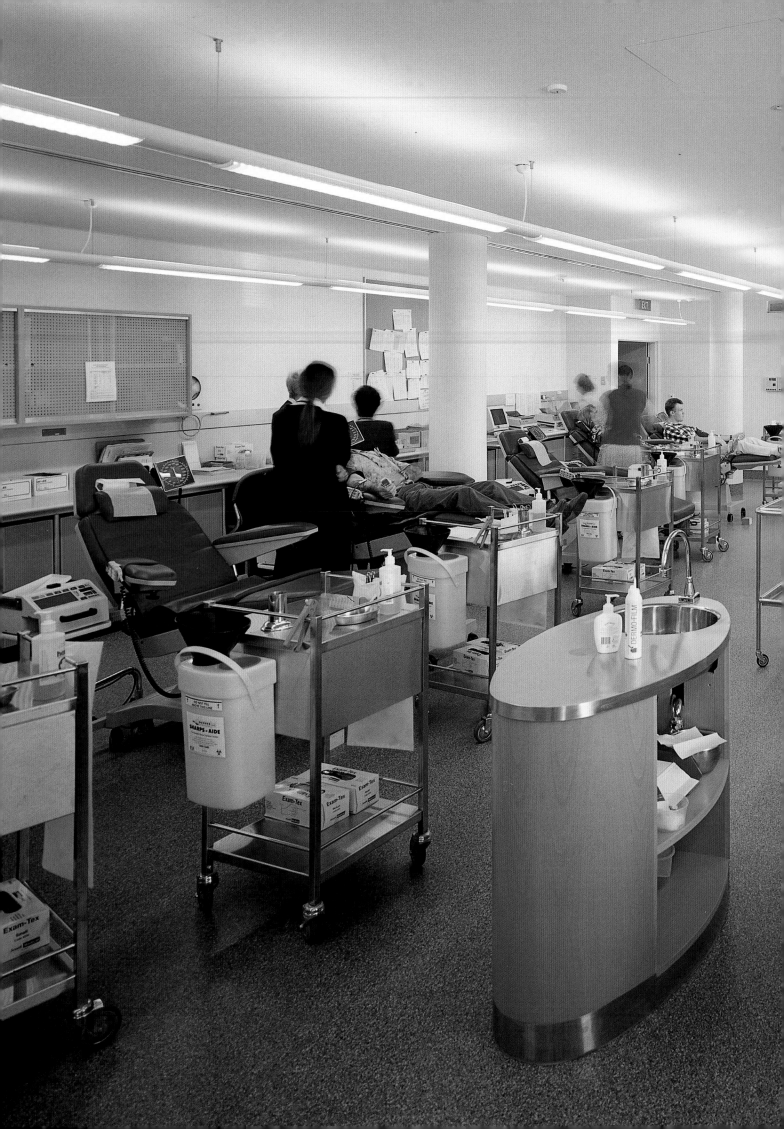

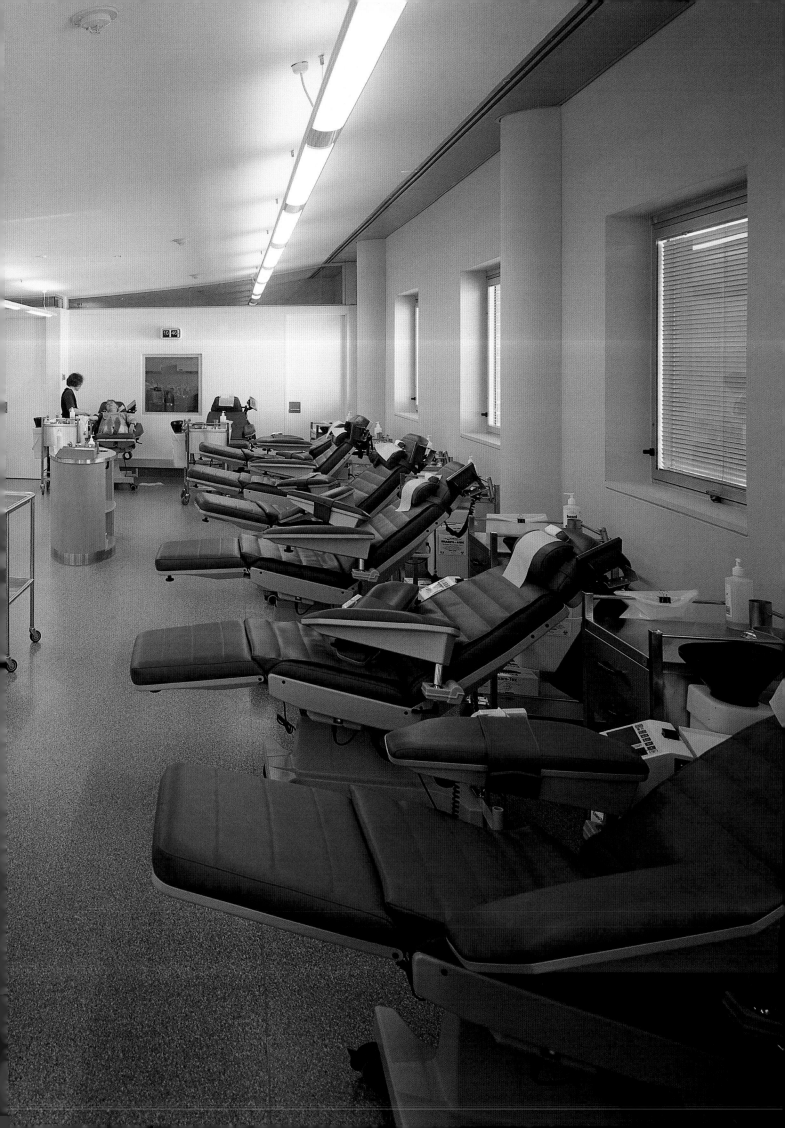

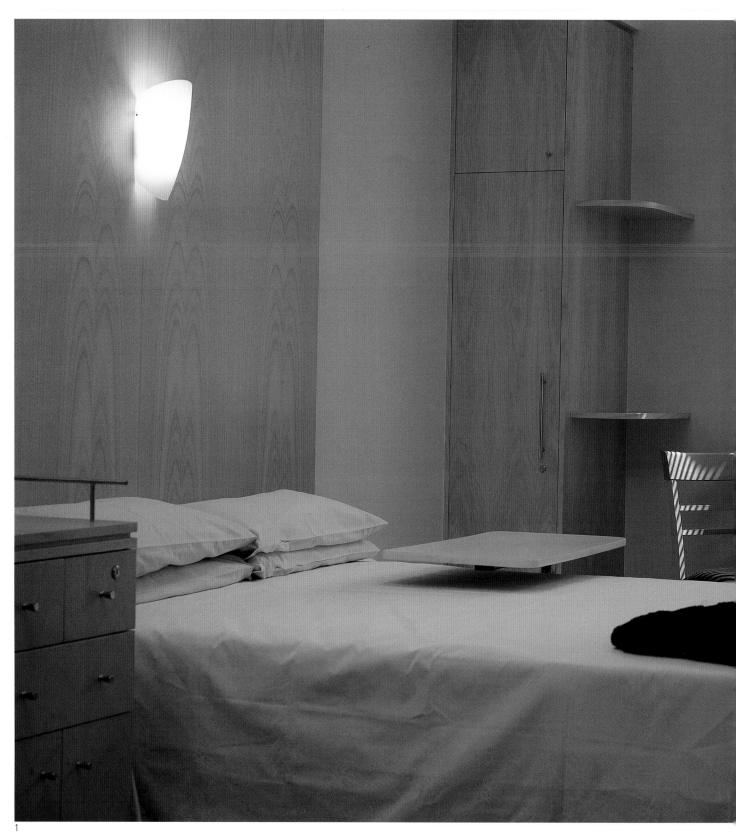

1

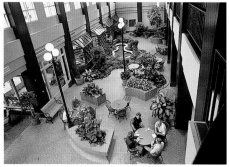

2

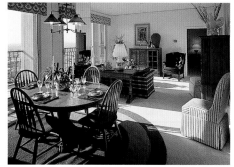

3

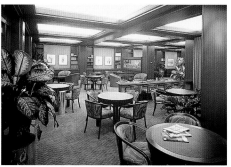

4

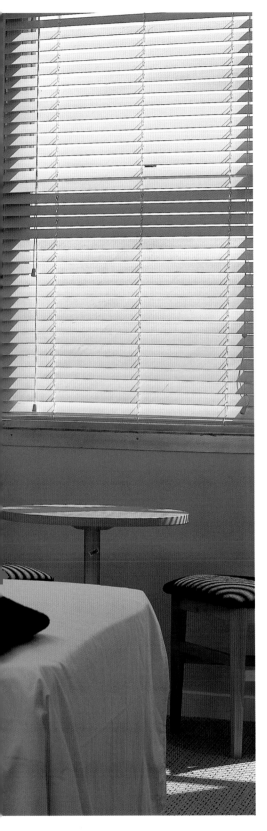

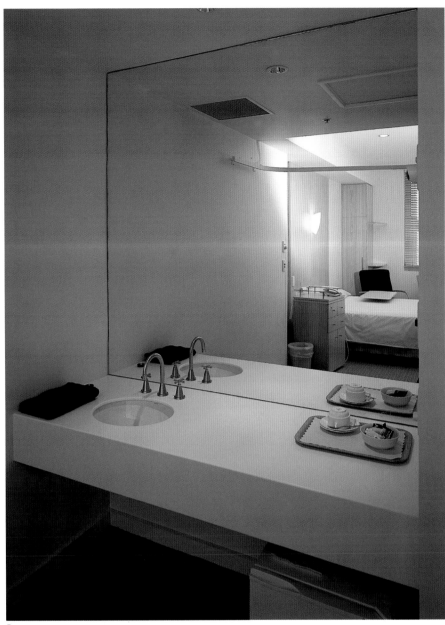

5

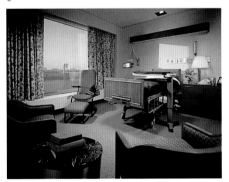

6

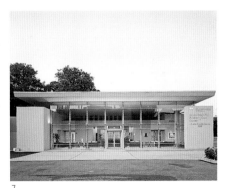

7

Frances Perry Private Hospital
Carlton, Melbourne, Australia
Woods Bagot

1&5   Typical antenatal room
Photo credit: Stuart Curnow

USAA Healthcare Center
San Antonio, Texas, USA
HKS Inc.

2   Social gathering space
3   Living suite
4   Club room
Photo credit: Rick Grumbaum

Mitstein Pavilion, Presbyterian Hospital
Manhattan, New York, USA
Skidmore, Owings & Merrill LLP

6   Private patient room
Photo credit: courtesy of Skidmore, Owings &
Merrill LLP

Maimonides Medical Center,
Sheepshead Bay Primary Care Center
Brooklyn, New York, USA
Lee Harris Pomeroy Associates/Architects

7   Street entry view of main exterior façade
Photo credit: Christopher Lovi

**The Toronto Hospital University
Health Network
Toronto, Canada**
Hellmuth, Obata + Kassabaum, Inc.
1&2   Cardiac Catheterisation Laboratories
Photo credit: courtesy of Hellmuth, Obata +
Kassabaum, Inc.

**Hinsdale Hospital
Hinsdale, Illinois, USA**
Loebl Schlossman & Hackl
Opposite:
          Recovery room
Photo credit: Mark Ballogg, Steinkamp/Ballogg
Photography

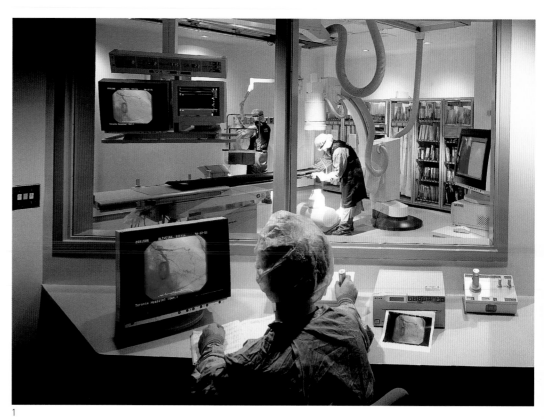

1

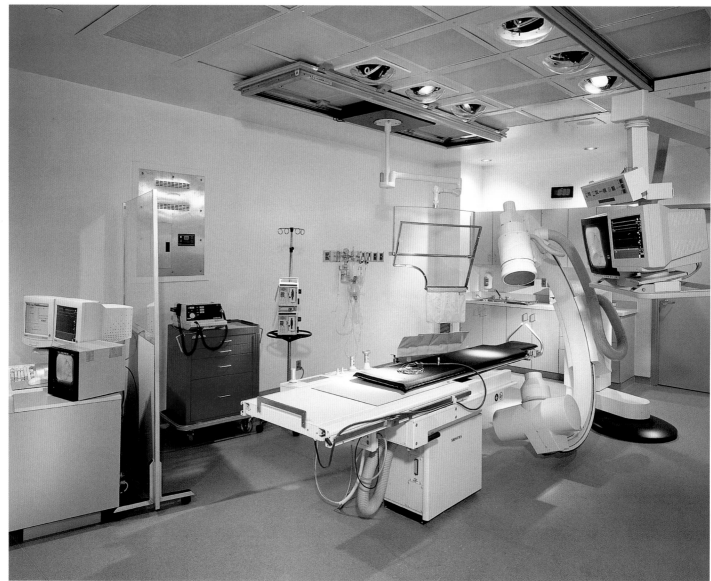

2

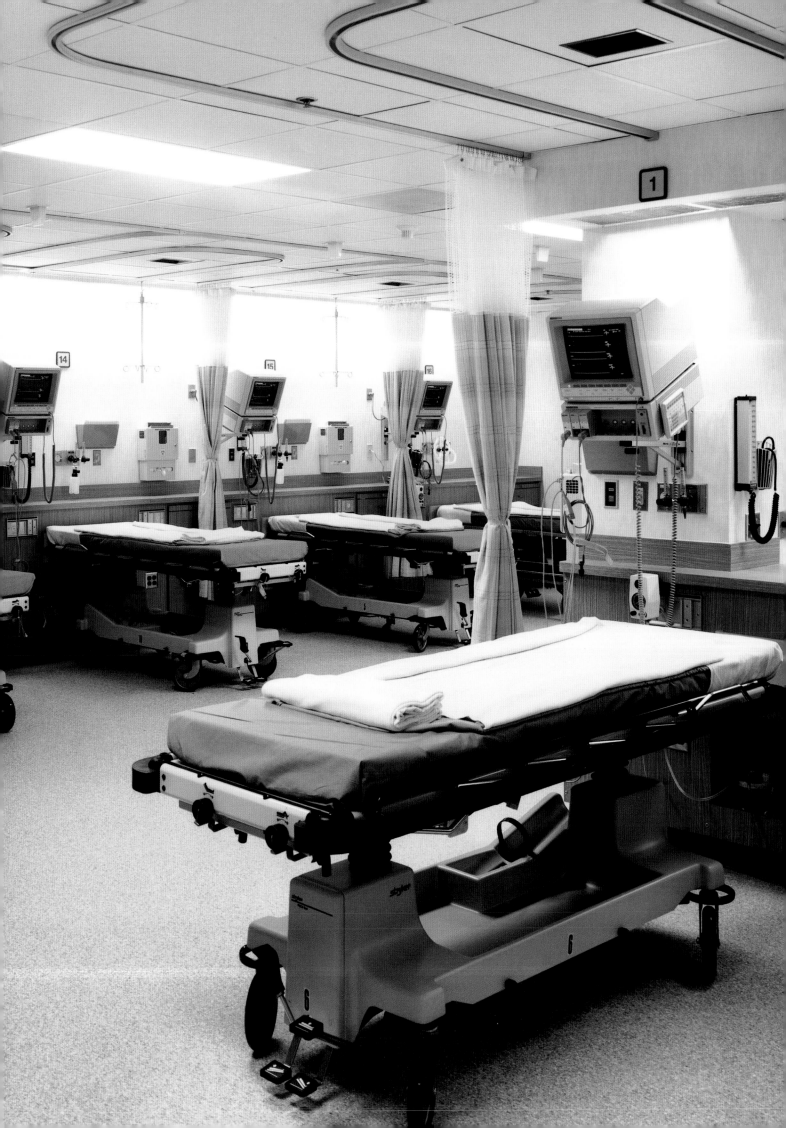

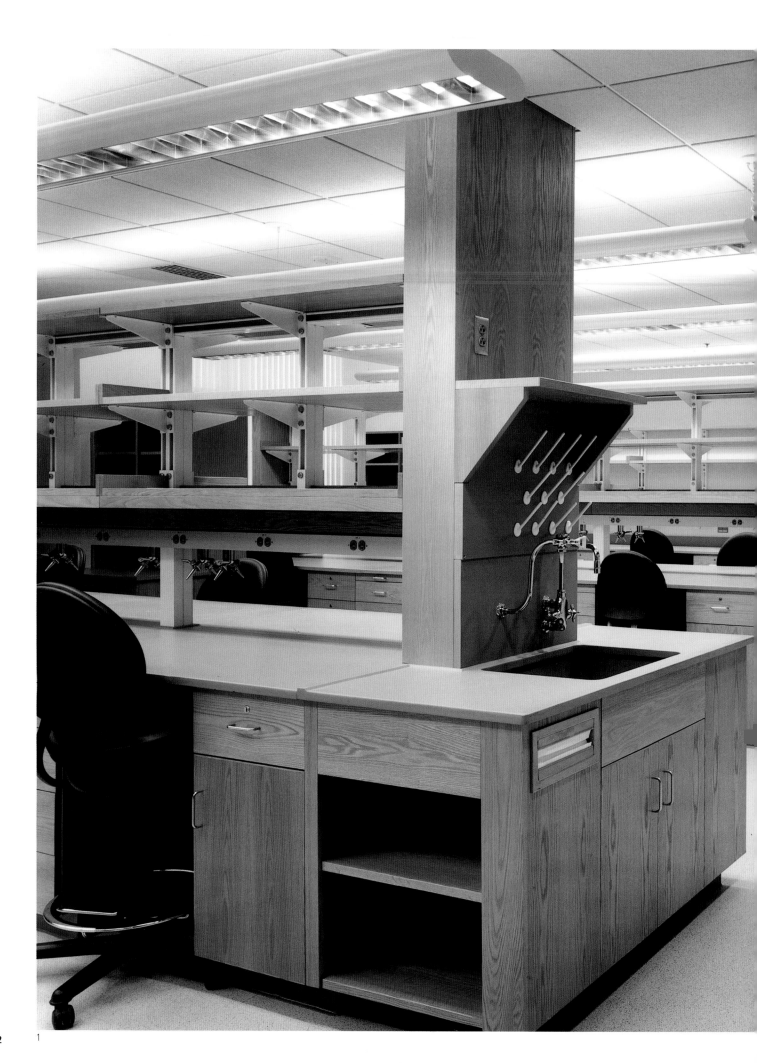

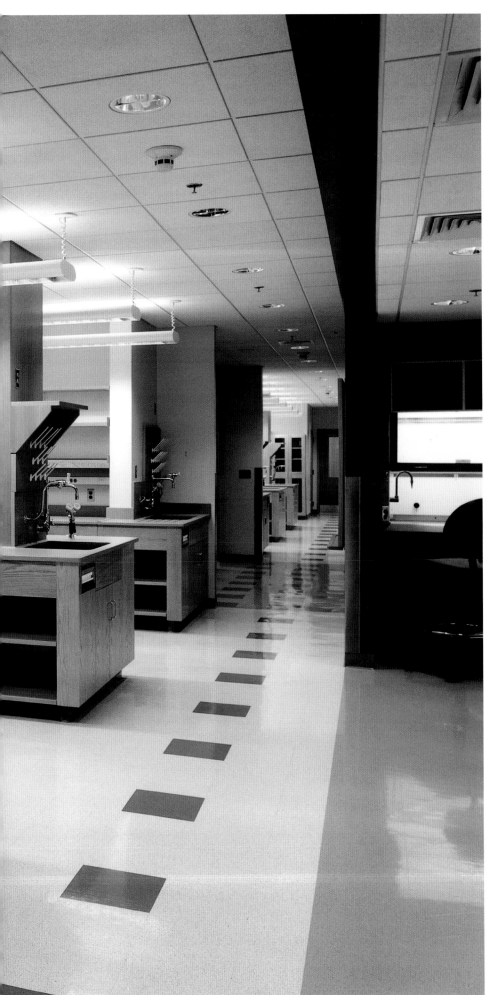

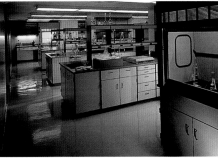
2

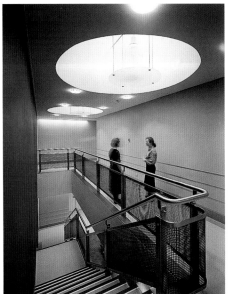
3

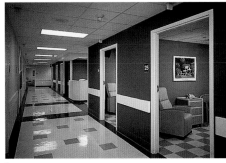
4

**Children's Hospital of Philadelphia,
Abramson Pediatric Research Center
Philadelphia, Pennsylvania, USA**
Ellenzweig Associates, Inc.
1   Typical laboratory
Photo credit: Tom Crane

**Eleanor Roosevelt Institute for Cancer Research
Denver, Colorado, USA**
Davis Partnership P.C., Architects
2   Laboratory
Photo credit: courtesy of Davis Partnership P.C., Architects

**Blood Bank and Laboratories
Parramatta, NSW, Australia**
Ancher Mortlock and Woolley
3   Laboratory staff stair hall
Photo credit: Eric Sierins

**Northeast Georgia Health Services–
Short Stay Surgery
Gainsville, Georgia, USA**
Quantrell Mullins & Associates Inc.
4   Patient dayroom
Photo credit: Brian Robbins

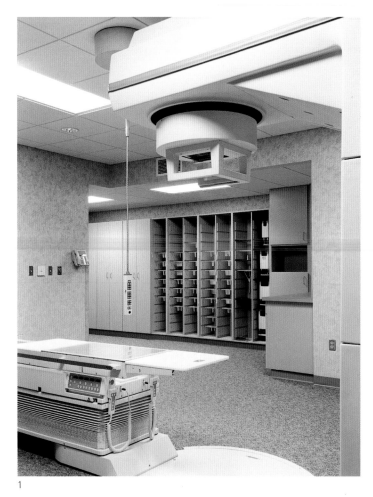

1

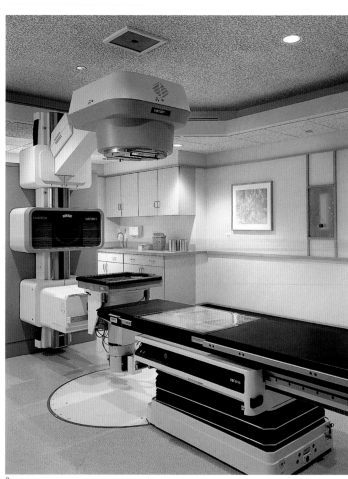

2

Barry Medical Park
Kansas City, Missouri, USA
WRS Architects Inc.

1   Linear Accelerator, heart of Radiation
     Oncology Suite
Photo credit: Mike Sinclair Photography

Evanston Hospital
Evanston, Illinois, USA
Loebl Schlossman & Hackl

2   Simulator room
Photo credit: Bruce VanInwegen

Alaska Native Medical Center
Anchorage, Alaska, USA
NBBJ

3   Exterior view of hospital
Photo credit: courtesy of NBBJ

Burton E. Green Child and Family
Development Center
California, USA
Barton Myers Associates, Inc.

4   Furnished benches at entrance for quiet
     conversations
5   Main entrance to lobby/reception area
6   Sheltered play space for four nurseries
7   Playground area leading from nurseries and
     atrium
8   Detail of garden showing exterior staircase
     to classroom
9   One of the nurseries seen from central
     atrium
Photo credit: Tim Griffith

West Suburban Hospital Medical Center
Oak Park, Illinois, USA
Loebl Schlossman & Hackl

10   Paediatric Department's reception area
     with rooms in background
Photo credit: Val Studio Photography

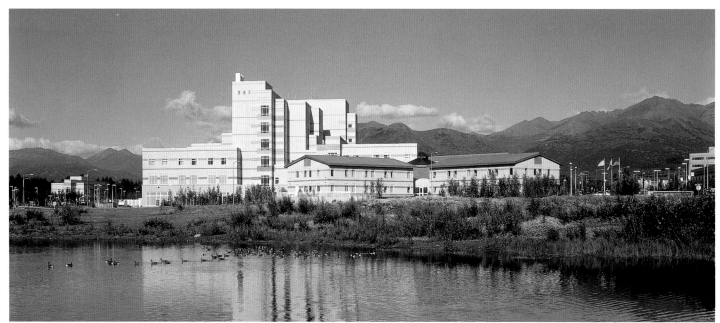

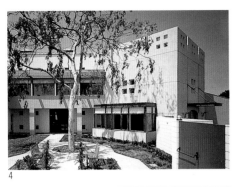

4

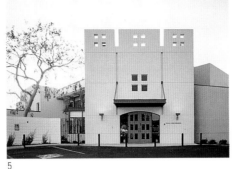

5

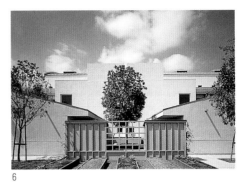

6

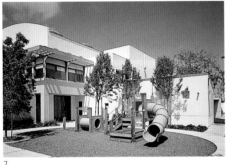

7

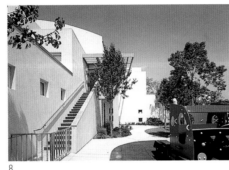

8

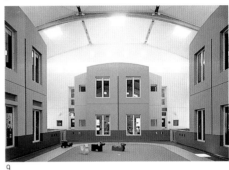

9

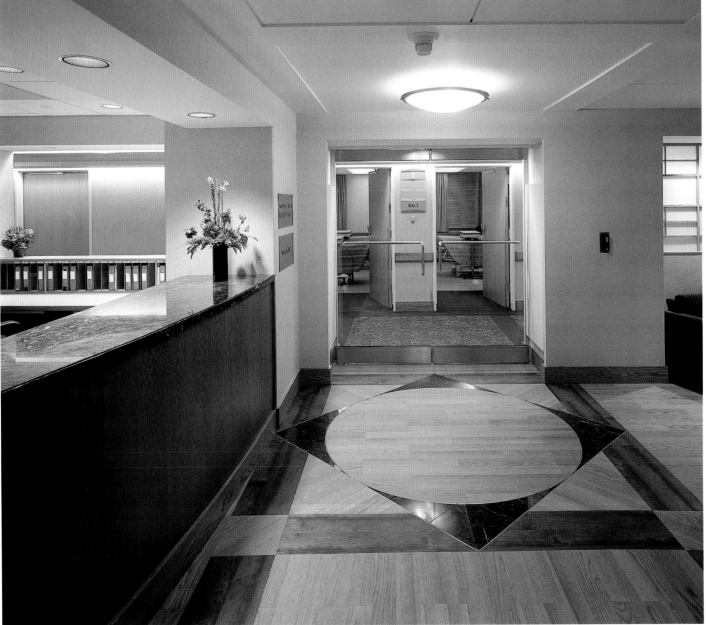

10

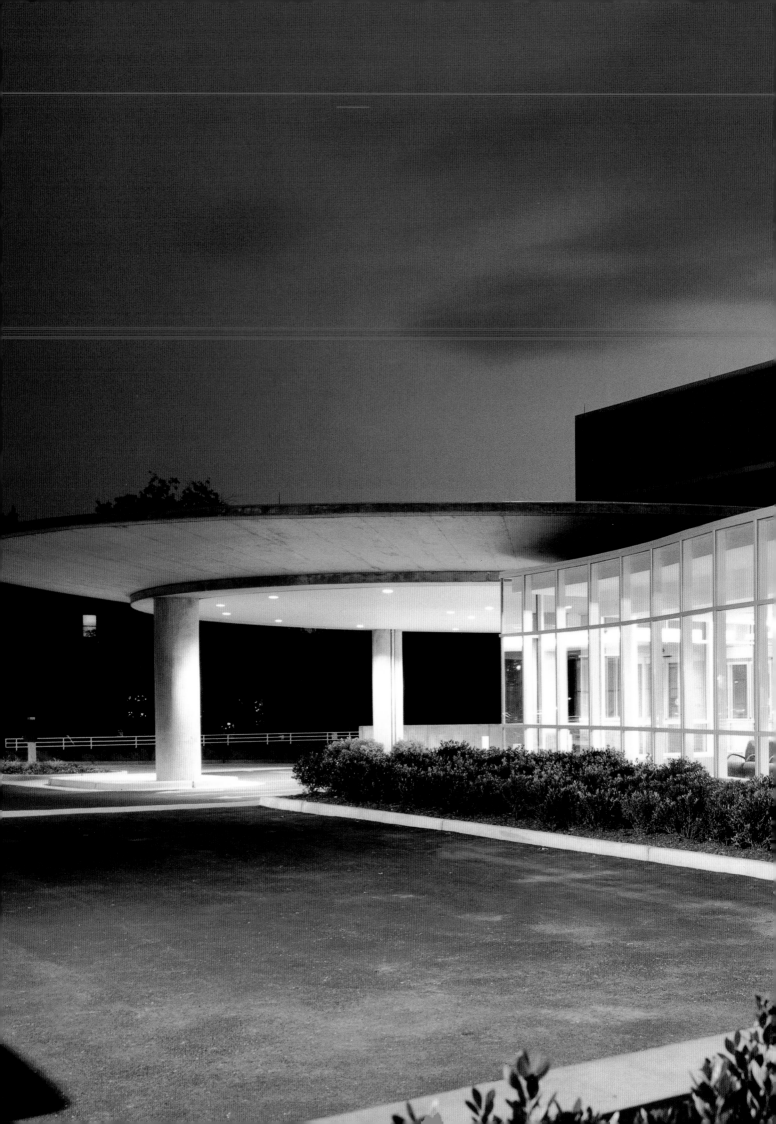

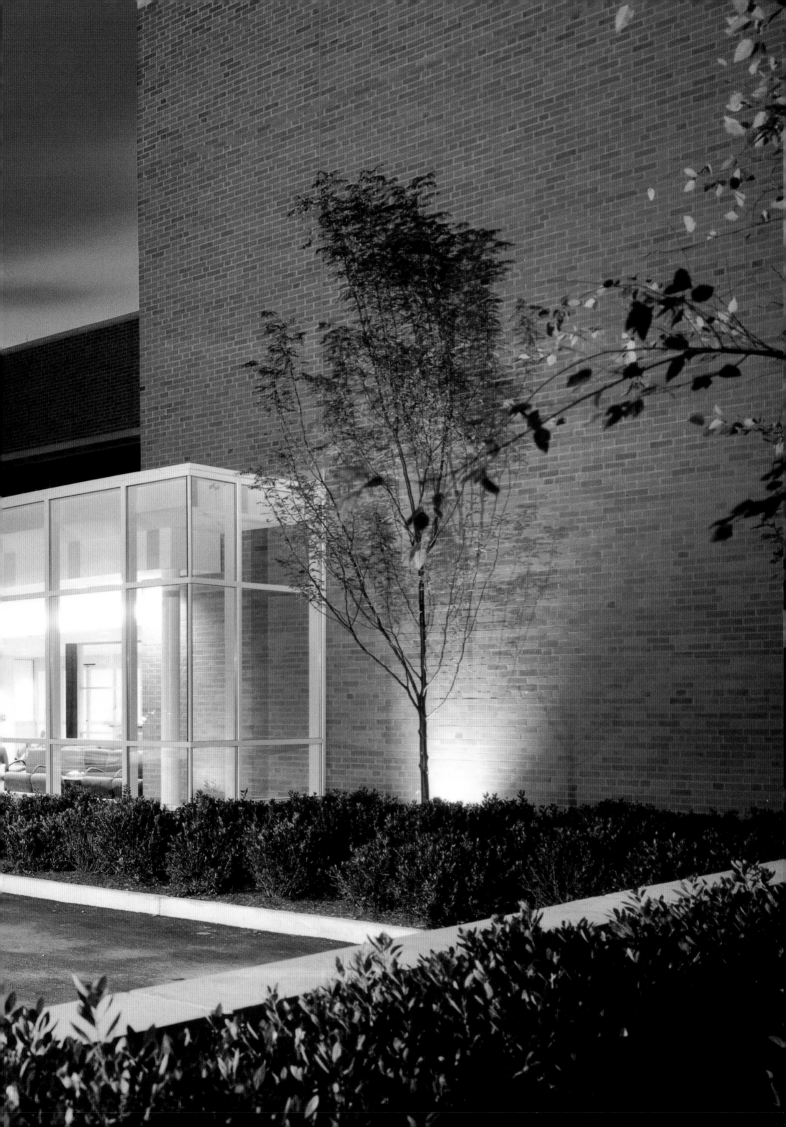

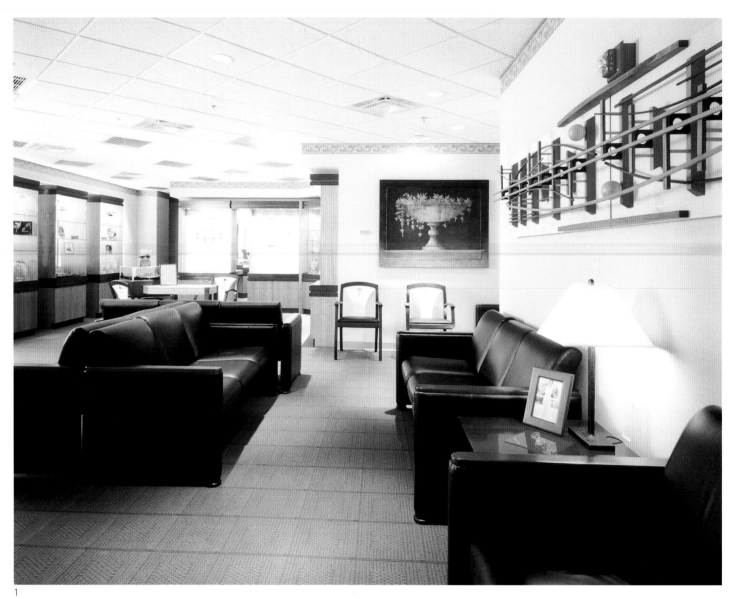

1

St. Mary's Health Center
Missouri, USA
Mackey Mitchell Associates
Previous pages:
    Circular entry canopy, defining shape for
    orientation
Photo credit: courtesy of Mackey Mitchell
Associates

Barry Medical Park
Kansas City, Missouri, USA
WRS Architects Inc.
1   Waiting and display area for Vision
    Correction Center
Photo credit: Mike Sinclair Photography

Utah Valley Regional Medical Center,
Women's and Children's Addition
Provo, Utah, USA
HKS Inc. in association with Design West
2   Wards in women's and children's
    addition
Photo credit: Ed LaCasse

Garvan Institute of Medical Research
Darlinghurst, NSW, Australia
Ancher Mortlock and Woolley
3   Atrium gallery acts as circulation between
    laboratory units
4   Typical research laboratory
Photo credit: Eric Sierins

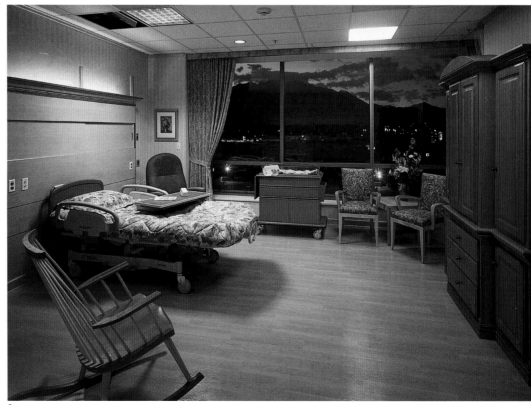

2

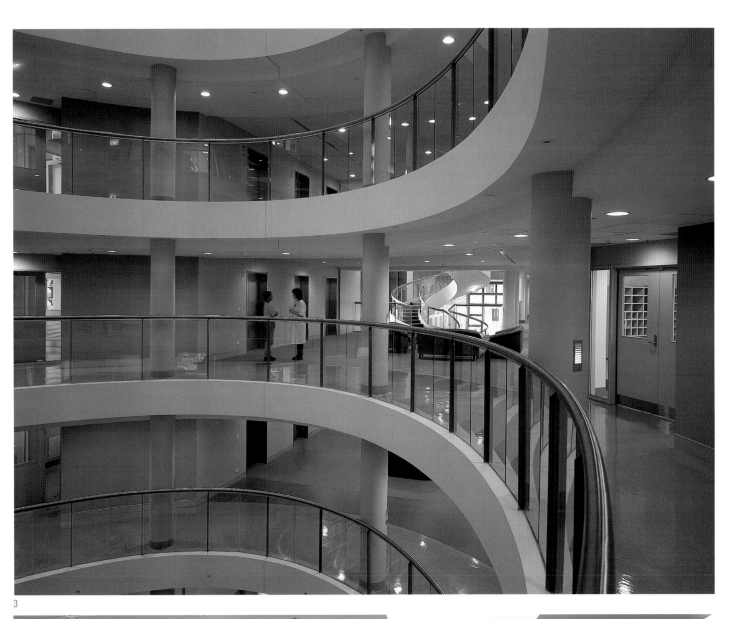

3

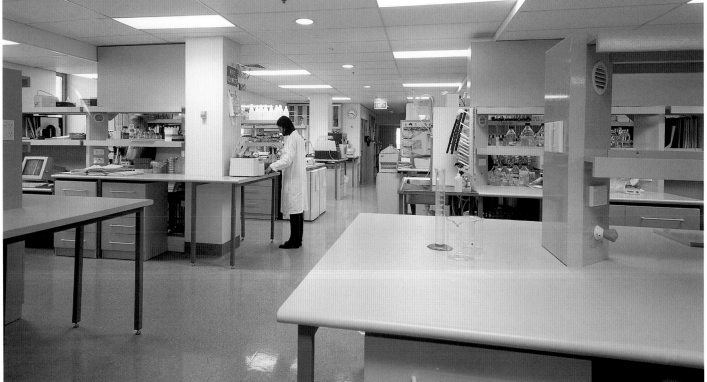

4

Swedish Medical Center
Seattle, Washington, USA
NBBJ
1 Ambulatory Care Center's recovery area
Photo credit: Assassi Productions

Lowell General Hospital,
Cancer Care Center
Lowell, Massachusetts, USA
TRO/The Ritchie Organization
2 Infusion treatment area
Photo credit: Edward Jacoby/Jacoby Photography

Prince of Wales Hospital
Randwick, NSW, Australia
Woods Bagot
3 Operating suite corridor
4 Endoscopy room
Photo credit: Bart Maiorana

University of Arkansas, Medical Sciences
and Biomedical Research Center
Little Rock, Arkansas, USA
WD & D/Wilkins & Sims/HKS Inc.
5 Public space
6 Research and laboratory commons space
7 Laboratory
Photo credit: courtesy of HKS Inc.

Littleton Hospital
Littleton, Colorado, USA
Davis Partnership P.C., Architects
8 Exterior view of hospital
Photo credit: courtesy of Davis Partnership P.C.,
Architects

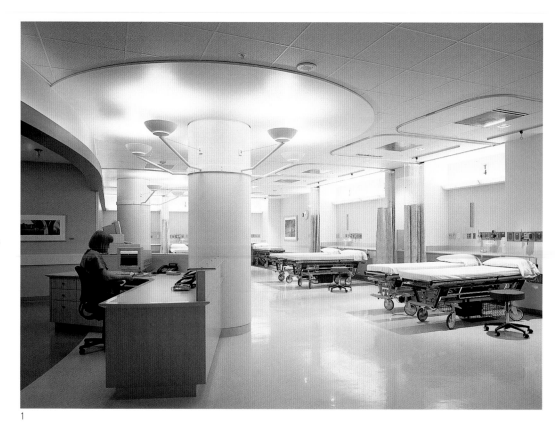

1

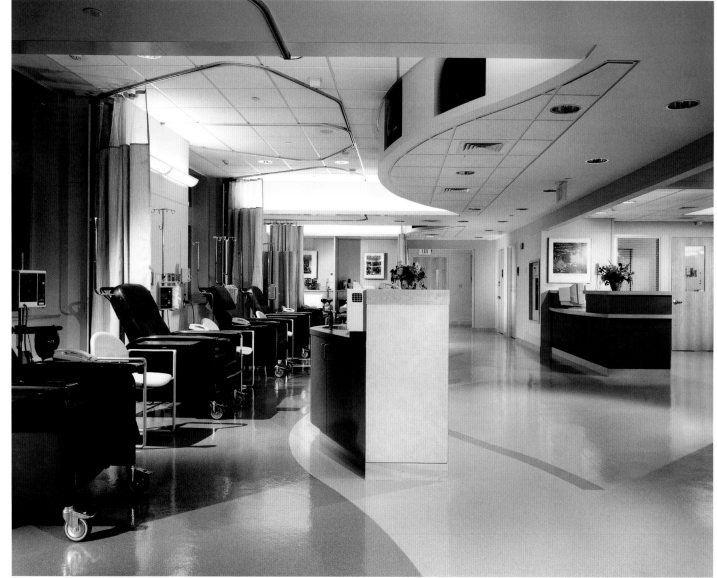

2

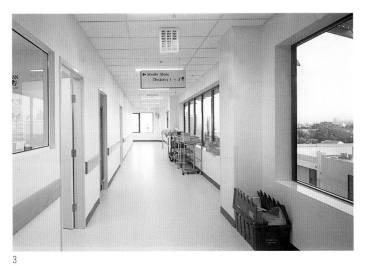

3

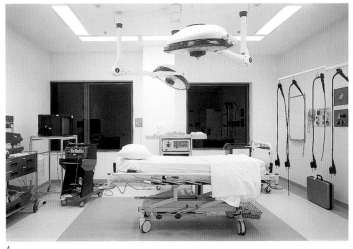

4

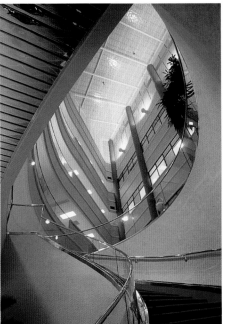

5

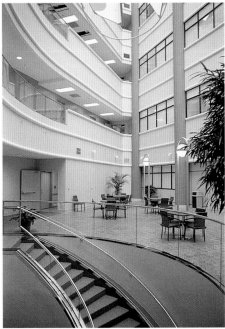

6

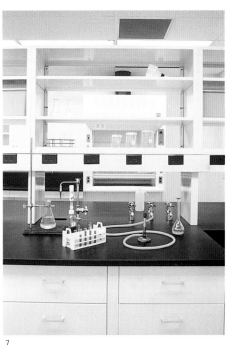

7

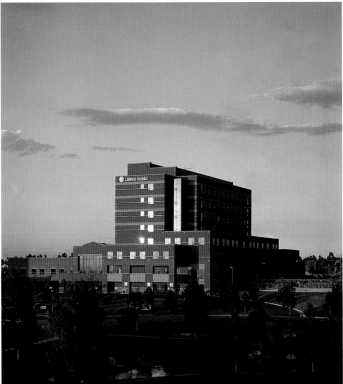

8

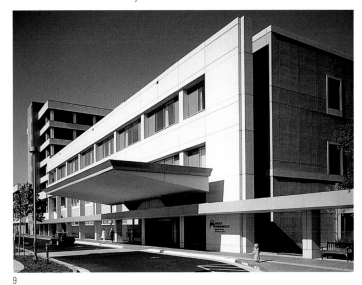

9

Kaiser Vallejo Hospital
Vallejo, California, USA
Skidmore, Owings & Merrill LLP

9   Main entry
Photo credit: courtesy of Skidmore, Owings &
Merrill LLP

Sutter Santa Cruz Maternity and Surgical
Center
Santa Cruz, California, USA
Kaplan McLaughlin Diaz in association
with Silva Strong Architects

Following pages:
    Birthing and surgical recovery suites along
    18-foot-wide corridors
Photo credit: Erich Anset Koyama

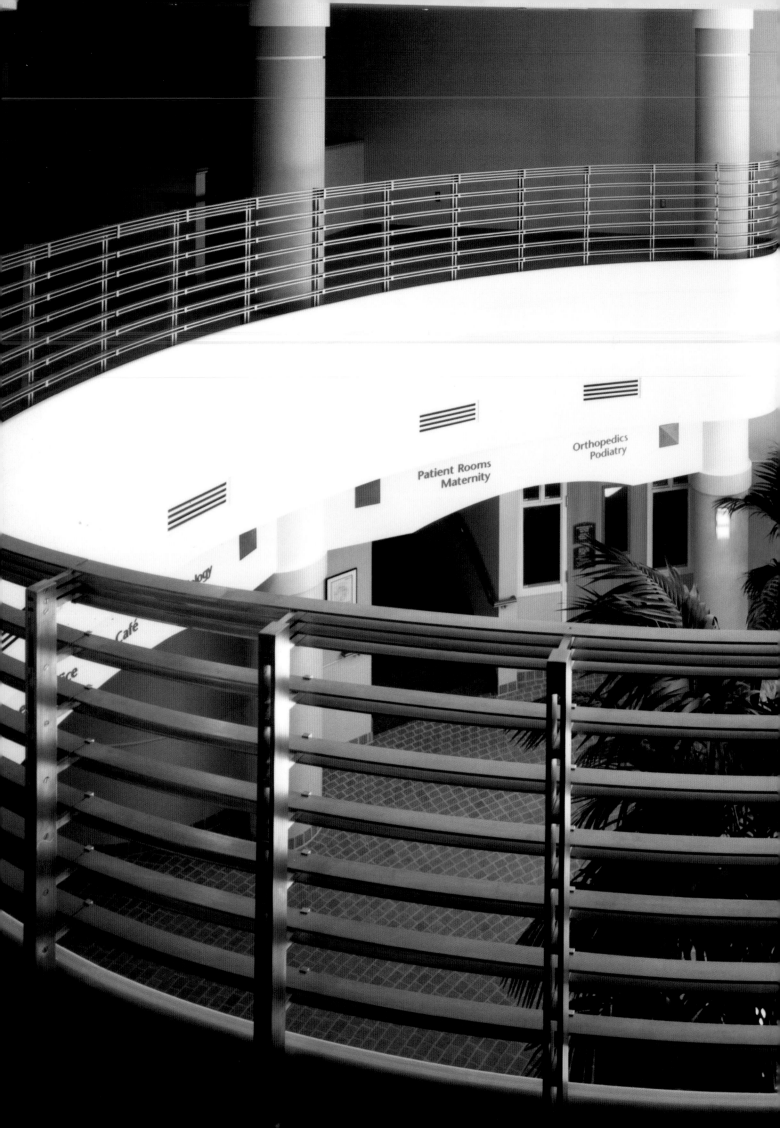

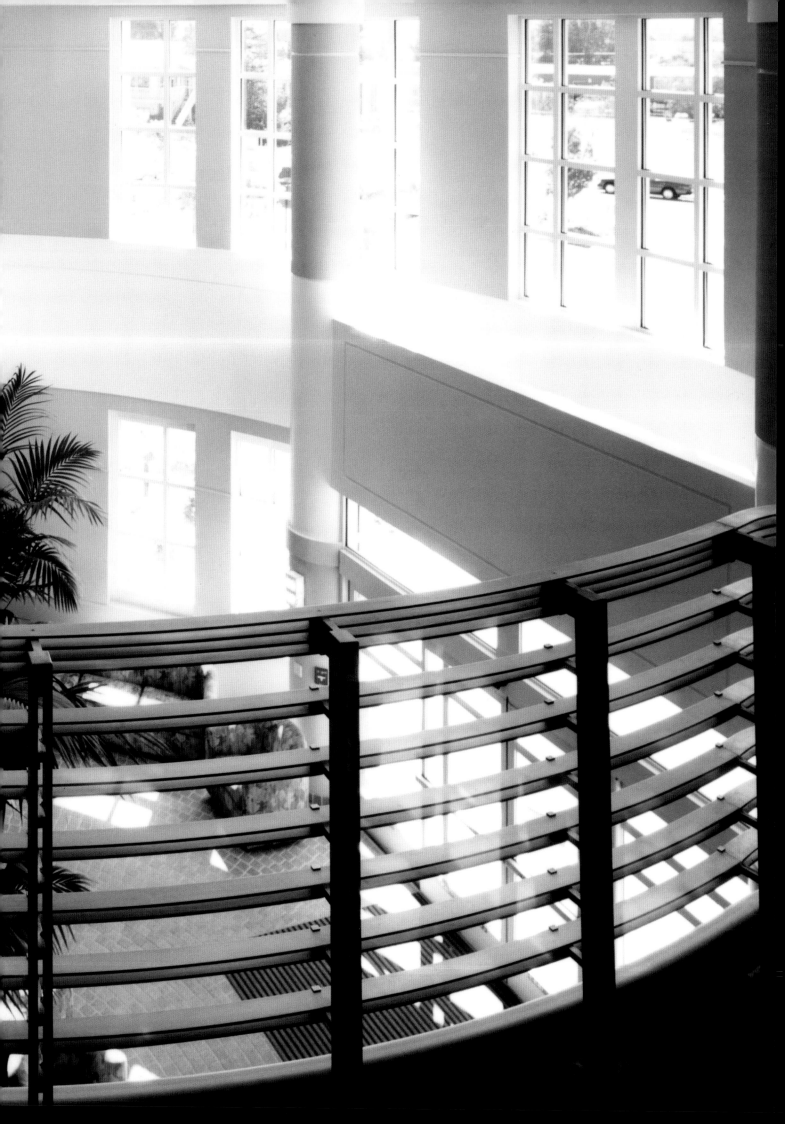

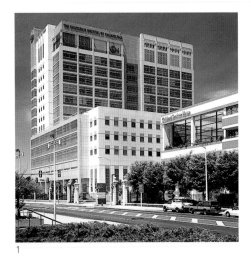

1

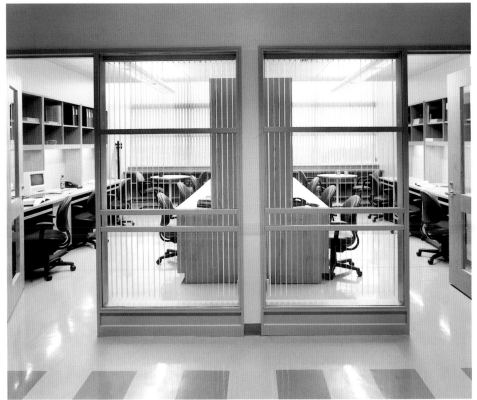

**Children's Hospital of Philadelphia,
Abramson Pediatric Research Center
Philadelphia, Pennsylvania, USA**
Ellenzweig Associates, Inc.

1   View from southeast
2   Desk room
3   Conference facilities
4   Cafeteria
5   Reading room
6   Conference room
Photo credit: Tom Crane

2

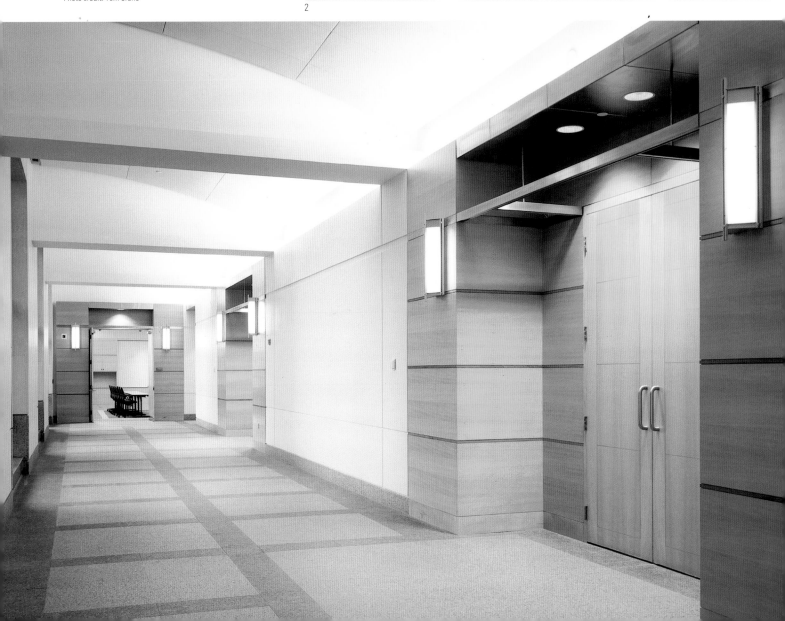

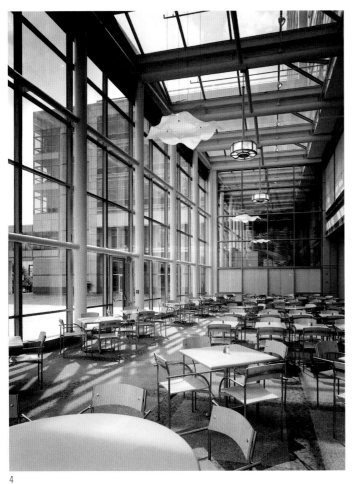

4

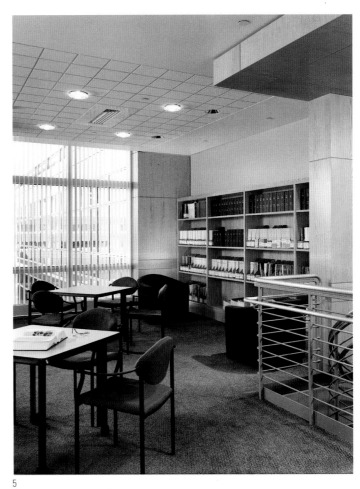

5

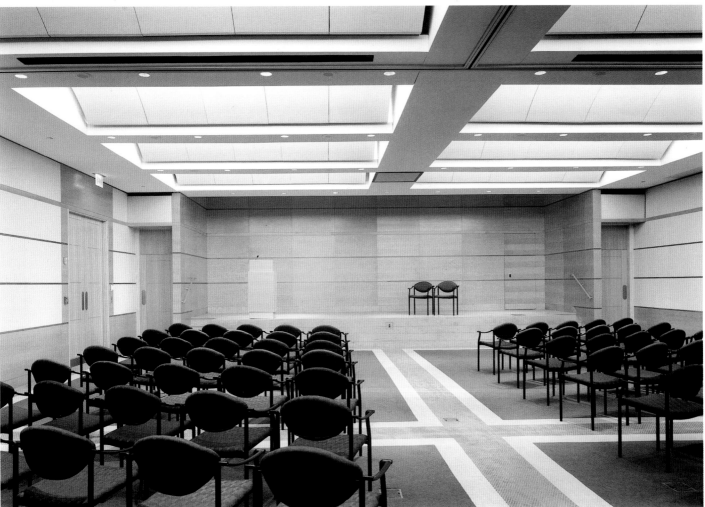

6

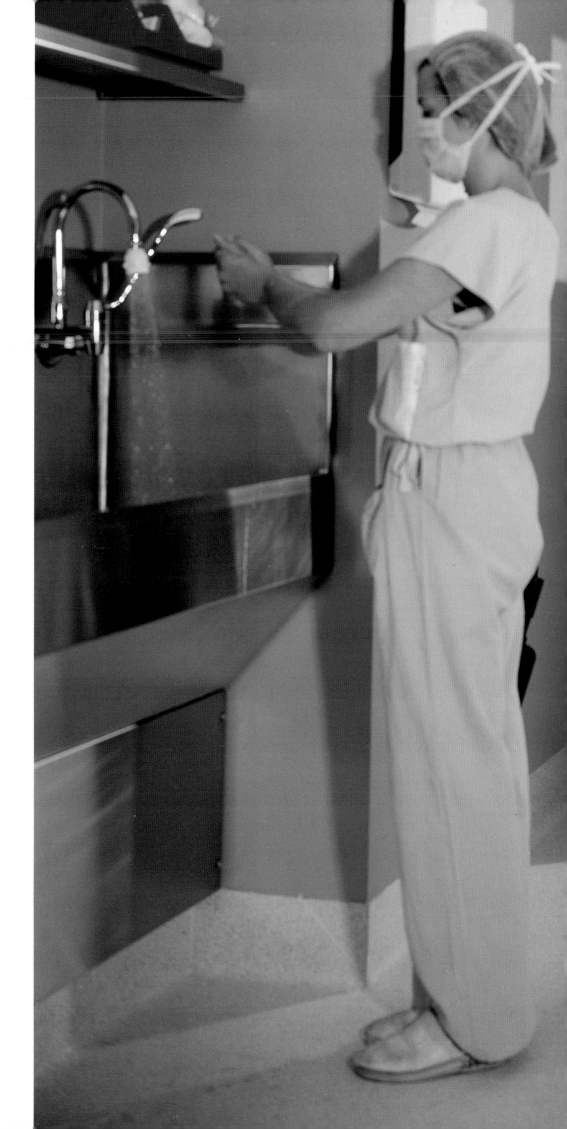

Frances Perry Private Hospital
Carlton, Melbourne, Australia
Woods Bagot
View into operating room
Photo credit: Stuart Curnow

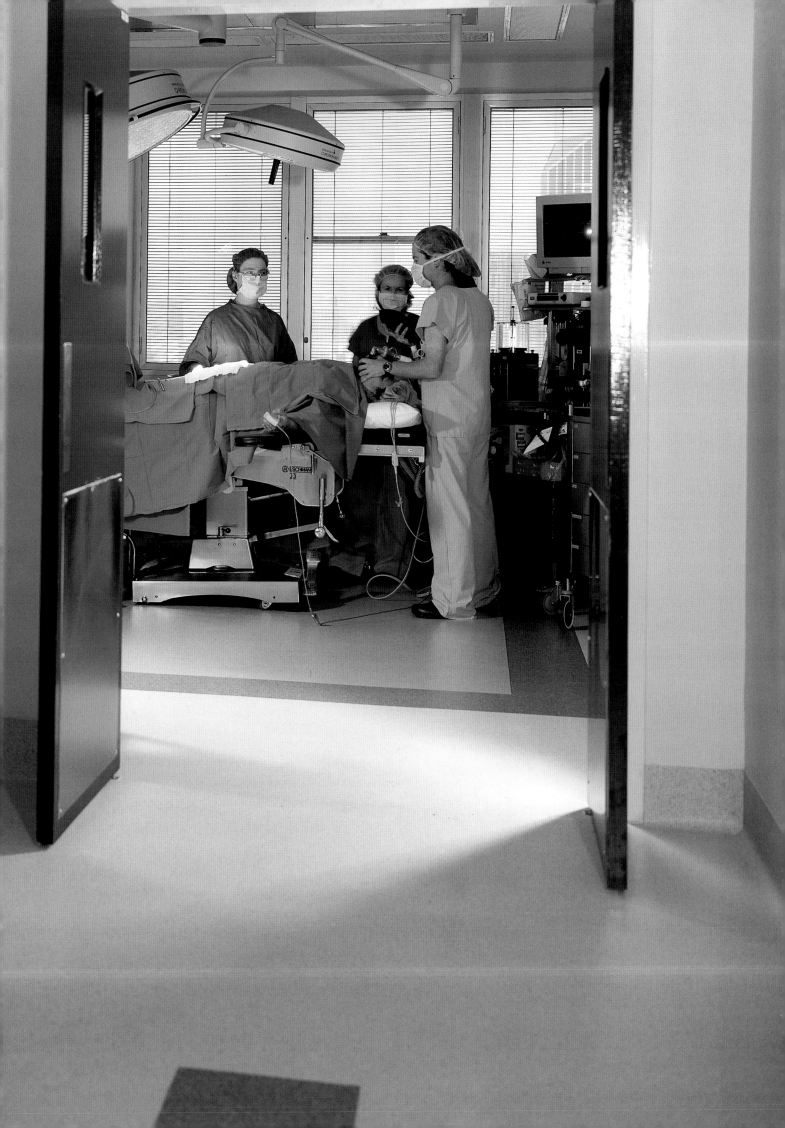

Patient and Family Learning Center,
Massachusetts General Hospital
Boston, Massachusetts, USA
The Stubbins Associates, Inc.
1   Entry off main corridor
2   Media Center with Internet access
3   Library overlooking Bulfinch lawn
4   Library with view to main reception area
Photo credit: Kevin Burke

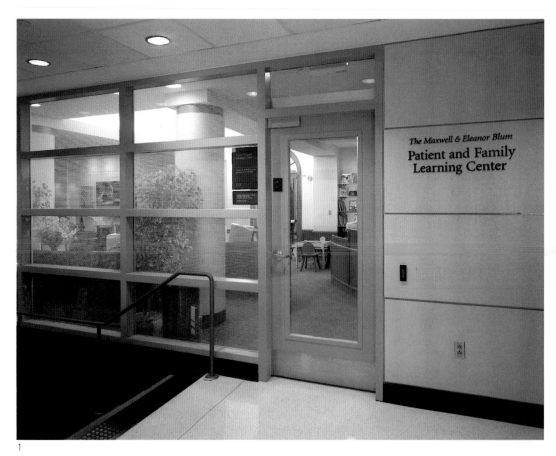

1

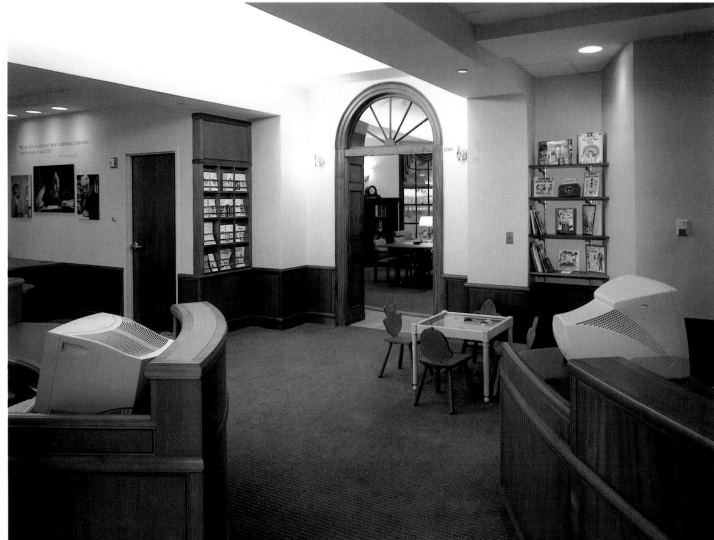

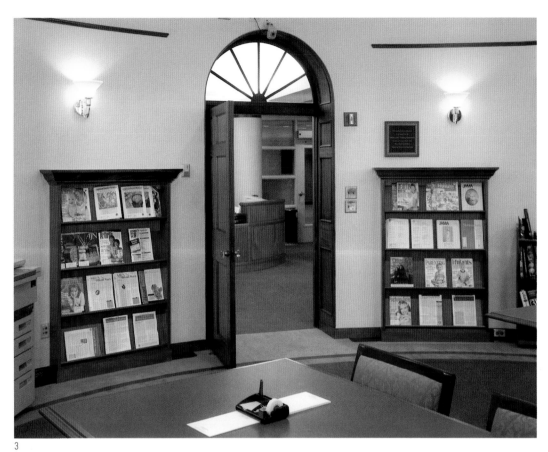

3

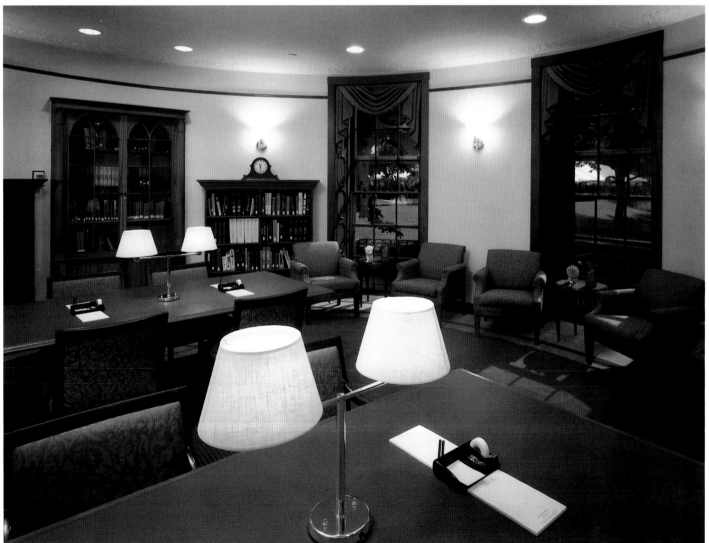

4

Northwestern Memorial Hospital
Chicago, Illinois, USA
Hellmuth, Obata + Kassabaum, Inc.
in association with Ellerbe Becket
1&2   Hospital offers advanced technology
        and flexible infrastructure
Photo credit: Craig Dugan/Hedrich-Blessing

Grossman Cancer Center,
Cancer Therapy & Research Center
San Antonio, Texas, USA
Marmon Mok
3   High energy linear accelerator vault
Photo credit: Aker/Zvonkovic

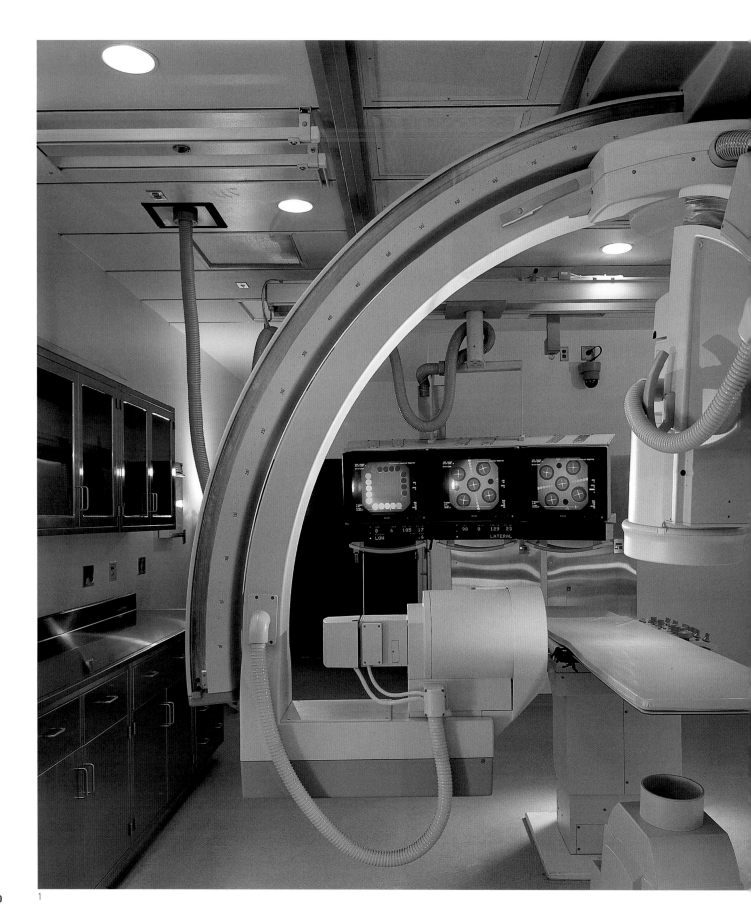

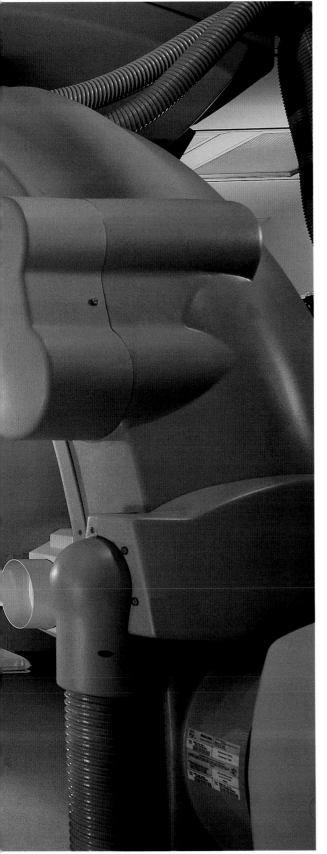

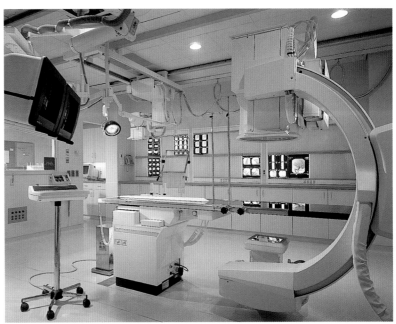

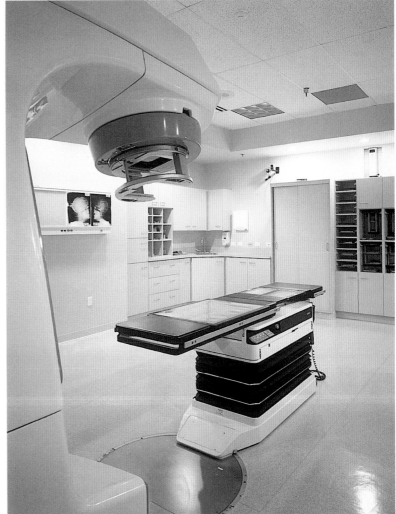

2

3

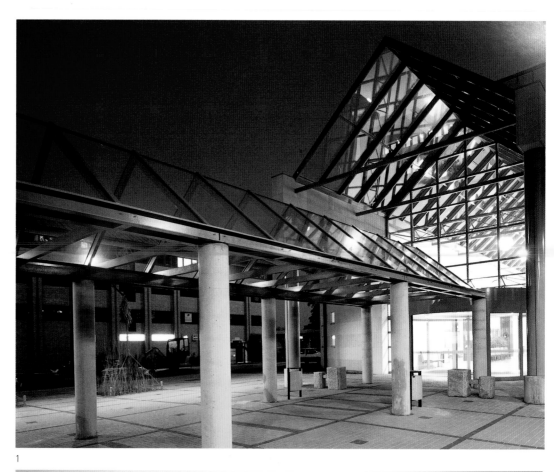

1

**Erasmus Hospital Addition
Brussels, Belgium**
Montois Partners

1   Exterior of reception hall and canopy
2   Reception desks
Photo credit: Marc Detiffe

**MD Anderson Cancer Center
Houston, Texas, USA**
LAN/HKS Inc. Joint Venture

Opposite:
    Public space
Photo credit: Rick Grumbaum

**Alaska Native Medical Center
Anchorage, Alaska, USA**
NBBJ

Following pages:
    Patient rooms take advantage of beauty
    outside
Photo credit: Assassi Productions

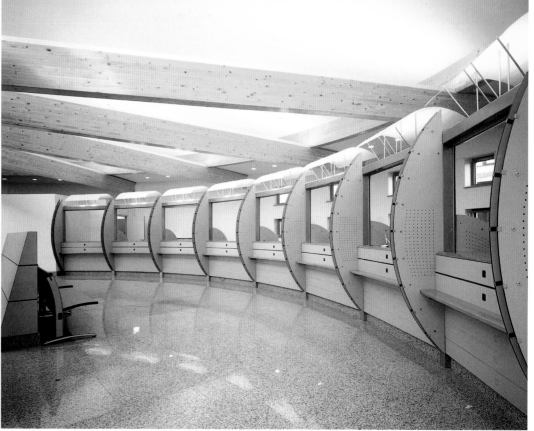

2

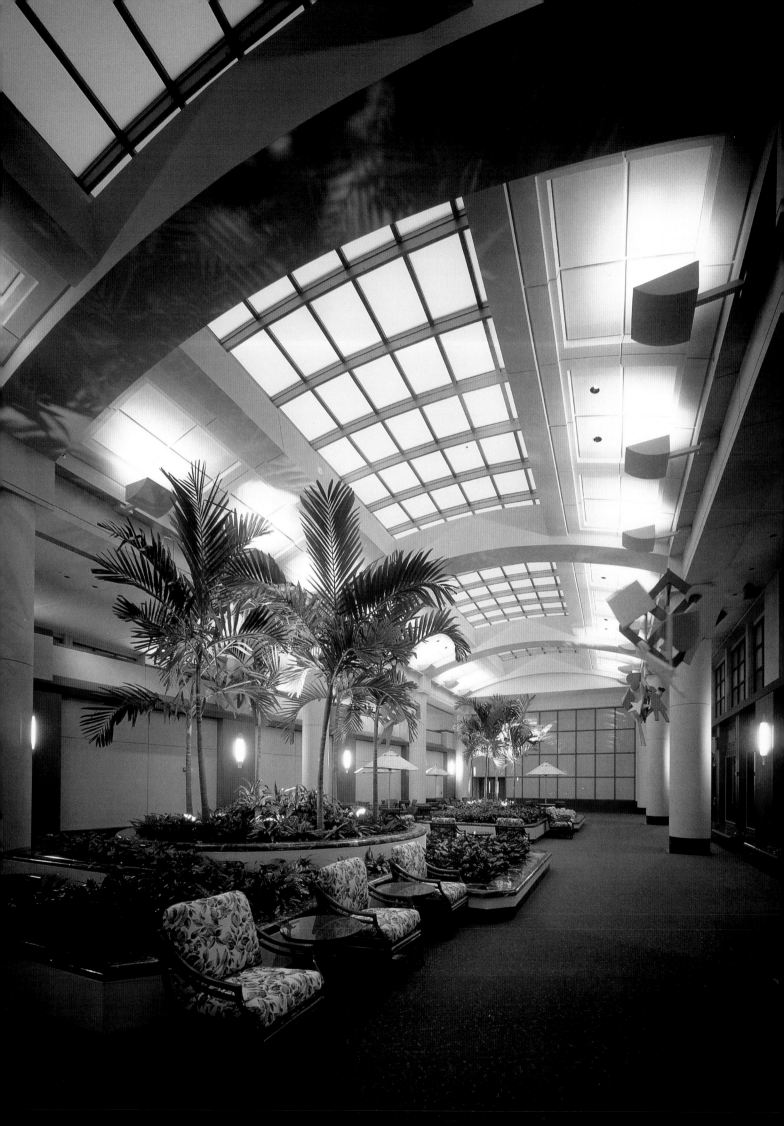

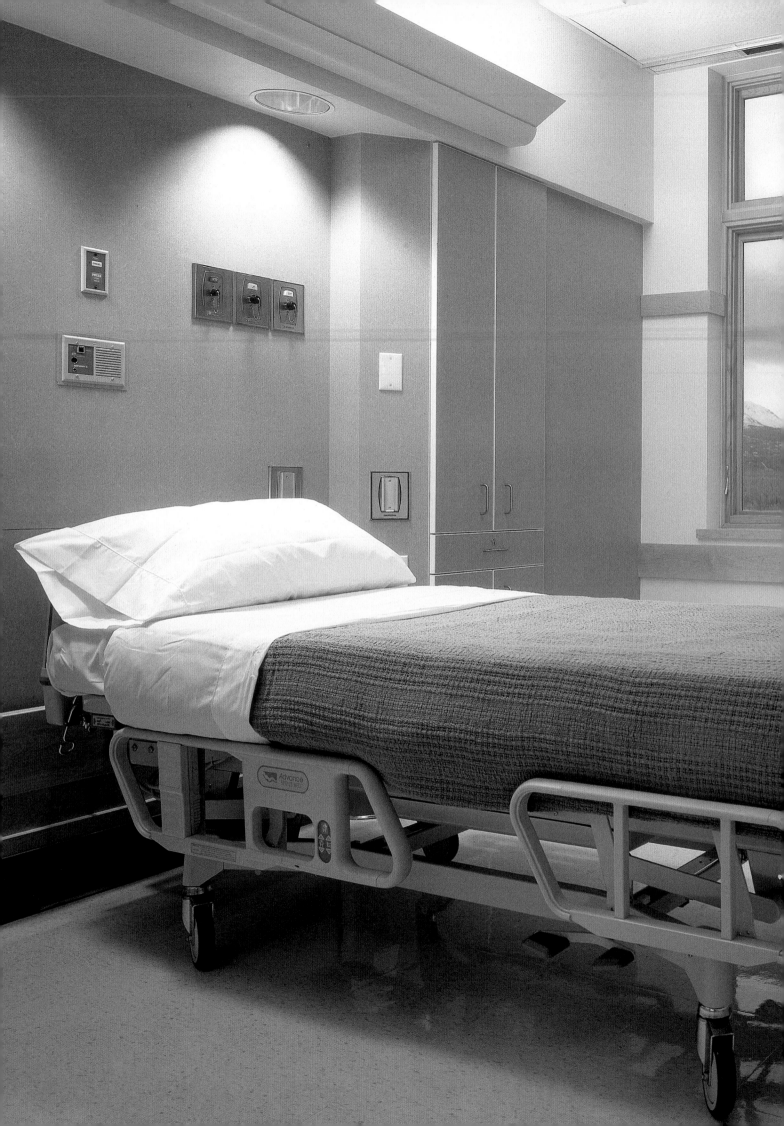

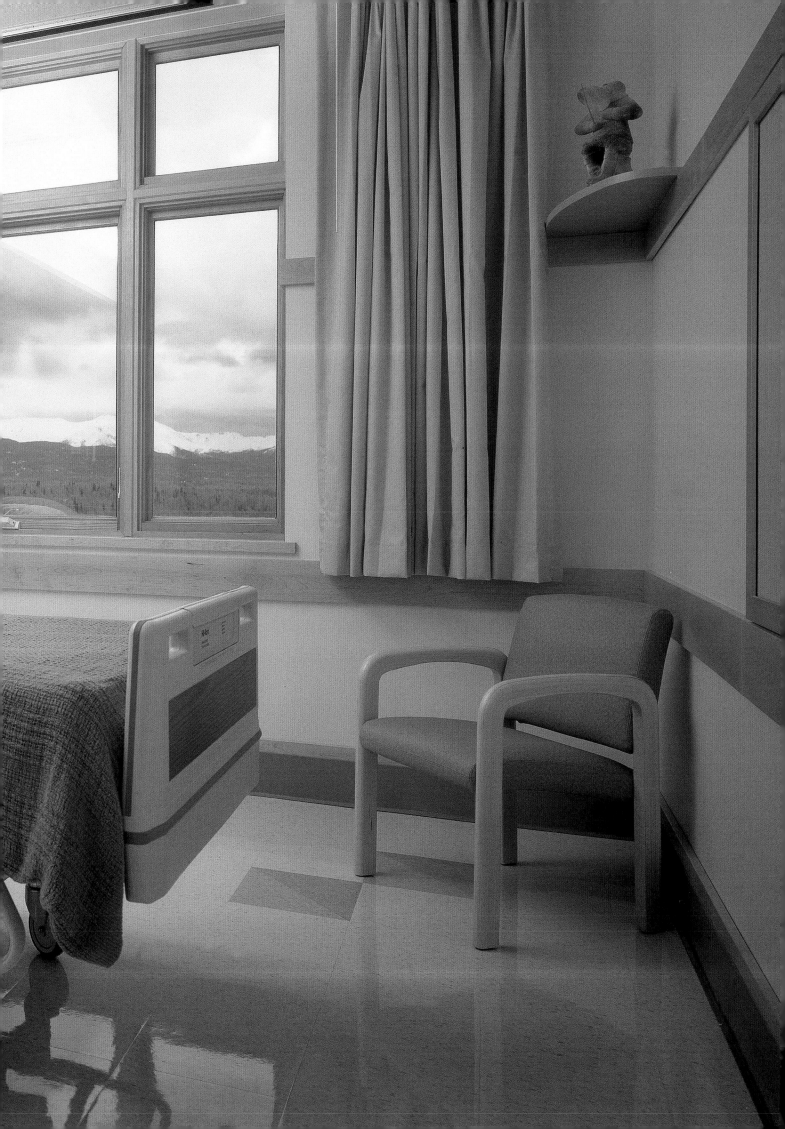

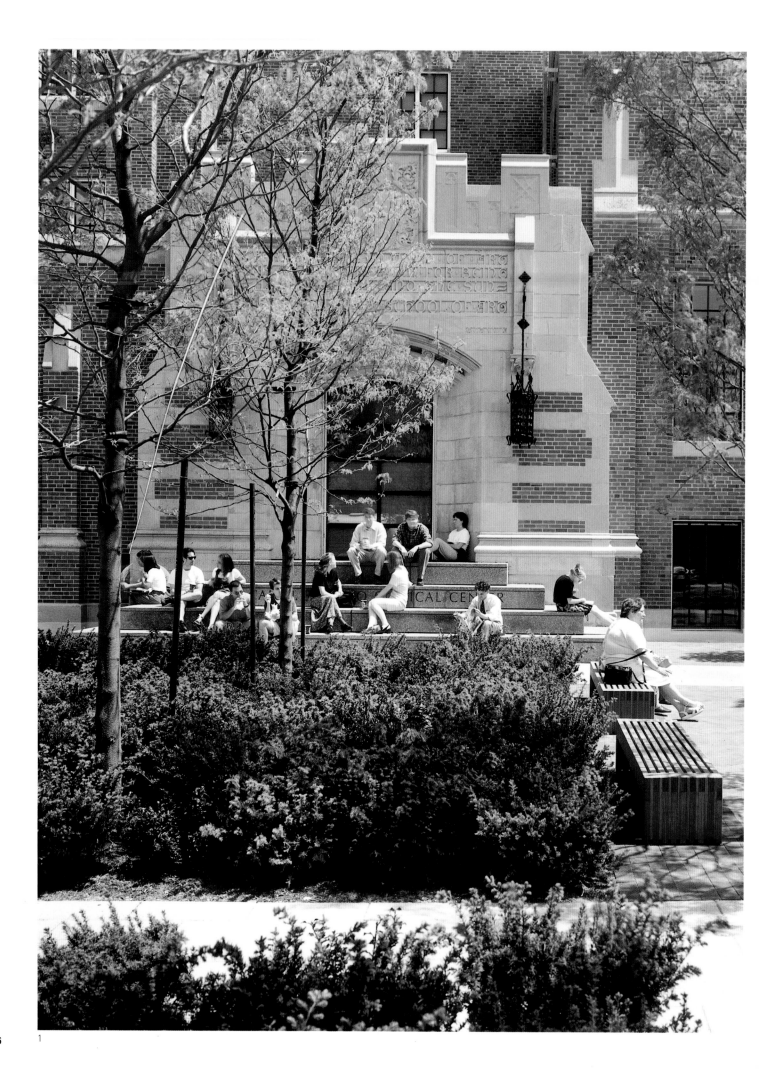

1

Carl J. Shapiro Clinical Center
Massachusetts, USA
Rothman Partners

1   Preserved historic façade, Brookline
    Avenue
2   Brookline Avenue façade and connector to
    hospital
Photo credit: Steve Rosenthal

Community Health Services
Connecticut, USA
Du Bose Associates, Inc., Architects

3   Patient services are arranged in a warm
    bright medical mall
Photo credit: Robert Benson Photography

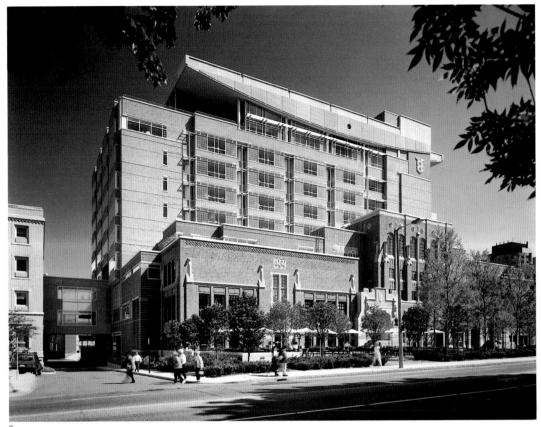

2

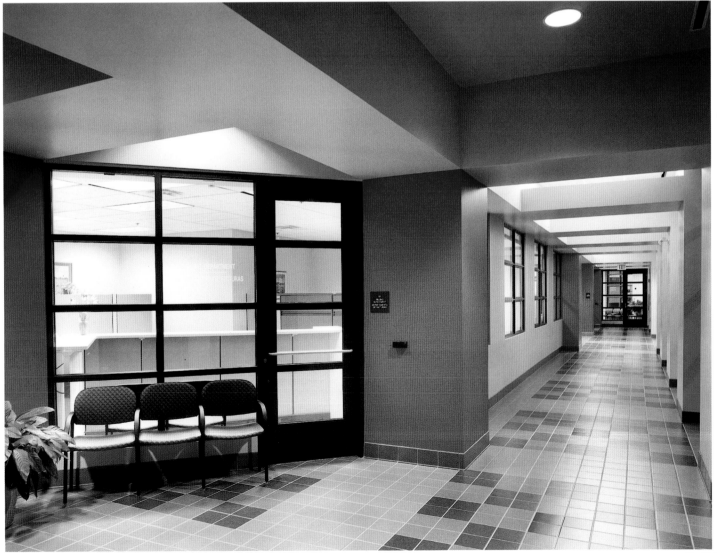

3

Prudential Health Care System HMO
Lithonia, Georgia, USA
Quantrell Mullins & Associates Inc.
1   Front entrance to Centre
Photo credit: Brian Robbins

Frances Perry Private Hospital
Carlton, Melbourne, Australia
Woods Bagot
2   Reception area
Photo credit: Stuart Curnow

University of Nebraska,
Lied Transplant Center
Omaha, Nebraska, USA
Hellmuth, Obata + Kassabaum, Inc.
in association with Leo A Daly
3   Children's play area
Photo credit: Paul Brokering

Avista Hospital
Louisville, Colorado, USA
Davis Partnership P.C., Architects
4   Foyer and waiting area
Photo credit: courtesy Davis Partnership P.C.,
Architects

Burton E. Green Child and Family
Development Center
California, USA
Barton Myers Associates, Inc.
5   Main reception area with inglenook
      and fireplace
Photo credit: Tim Griffith

Pomona Valley Hospital Medical Center
Pomona, California, USA
NBBJ
6   Exterior view of circular entrance and
      tree-lined boulevards
Photo credit: Hewitt/Garrison

Mayo Clinic
Rochester, Minnesota, USA
Payette Associates
7   Waiting area
Photo credit: Paul Ferrino

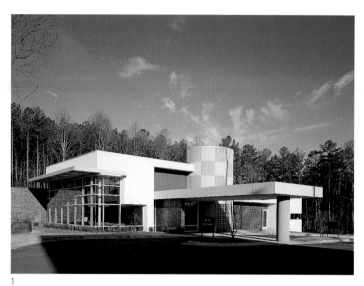

1

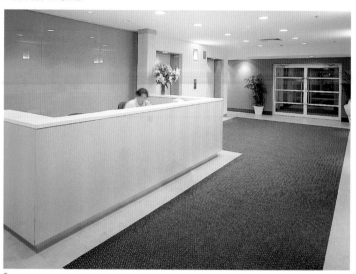

2

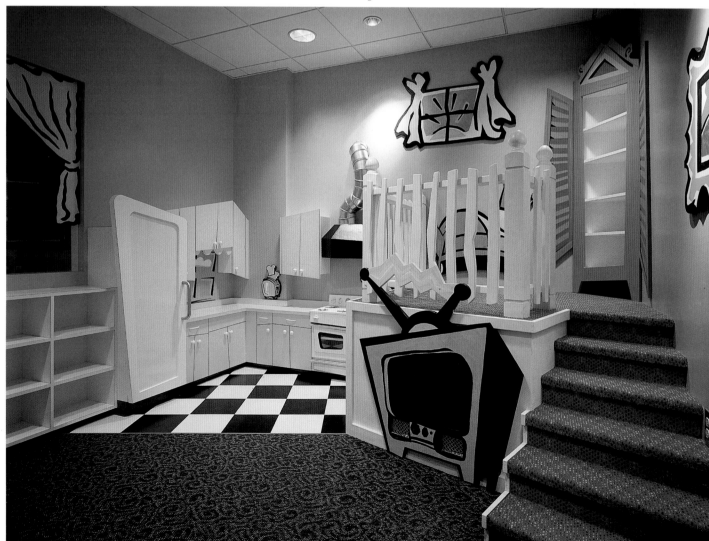

3

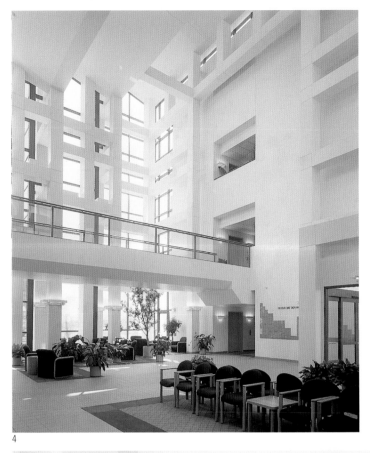

4

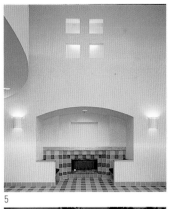

5

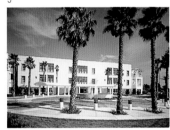

6

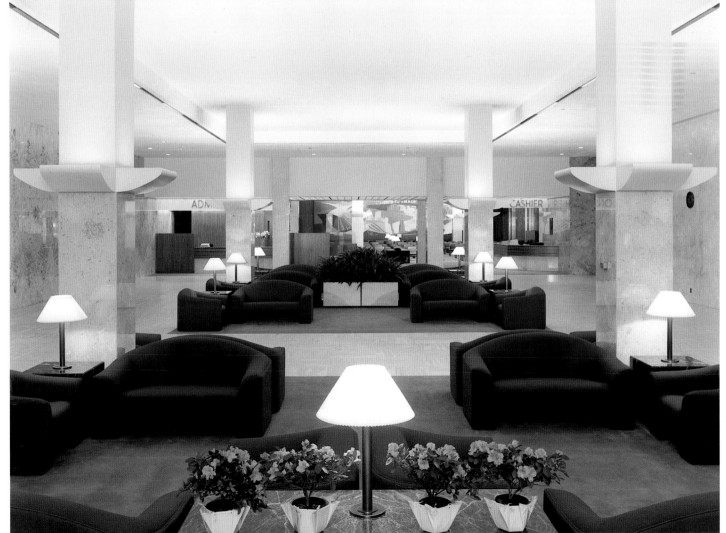

Gene Juarez Spa and Salon
Seattle, Washington, USA
NBBJ

1 Day Spa entrance with water feature
2 Upper level entrance gallery with cast
   glass wall
3 Day Spa corridor
4 Retail floor
5 Spa waiting area with water feature
6 Seating niche at entrance gallery
7 Spa treatment room
8 Vichy shower at Day Spa
Photo credit: Assassi Productions

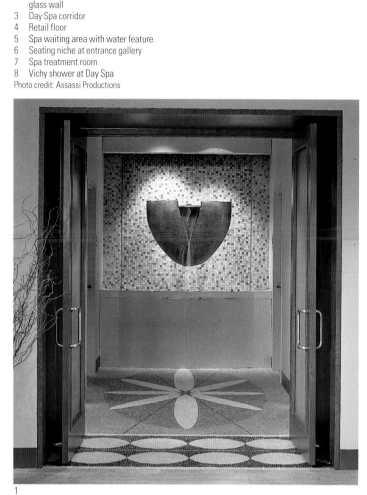

1

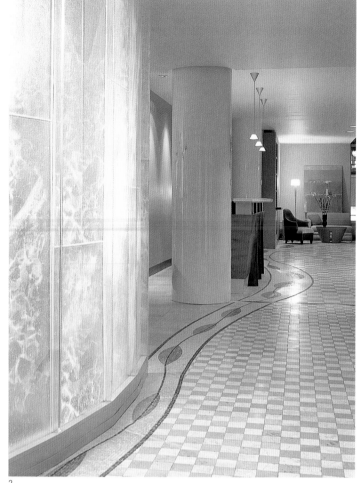

2

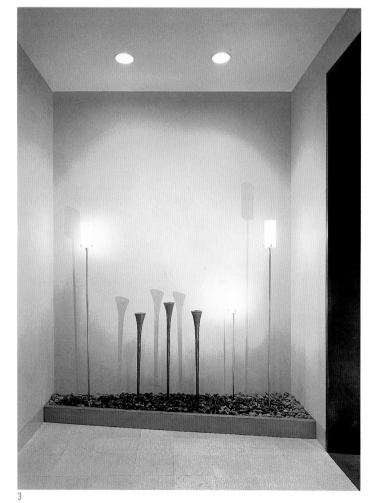

3

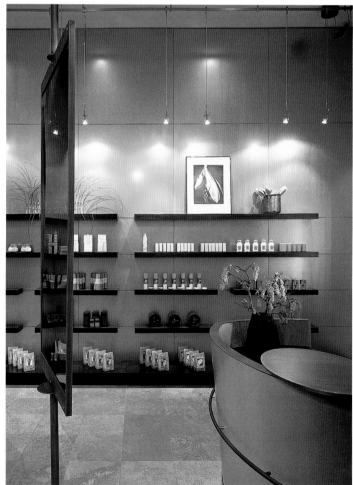

4

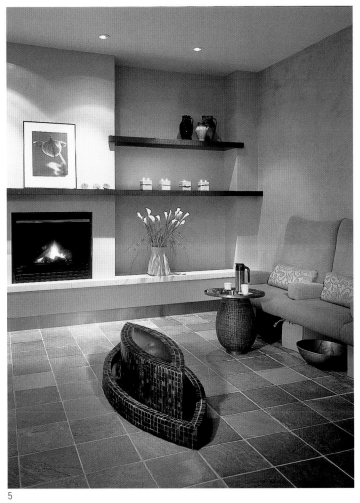

5

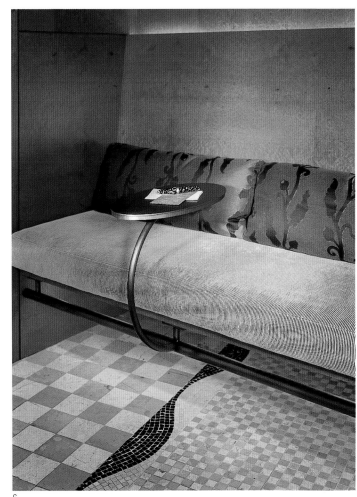

6

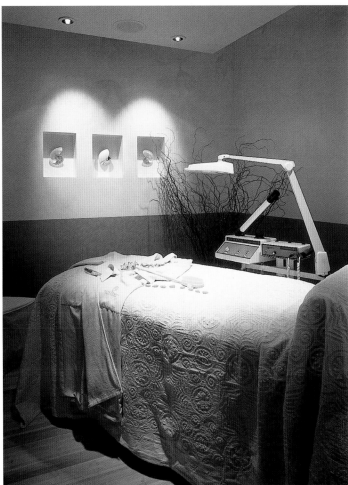

7

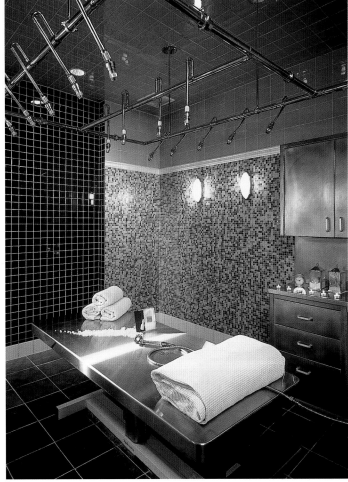

8

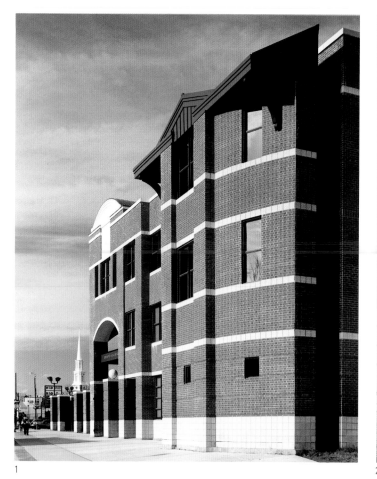

1

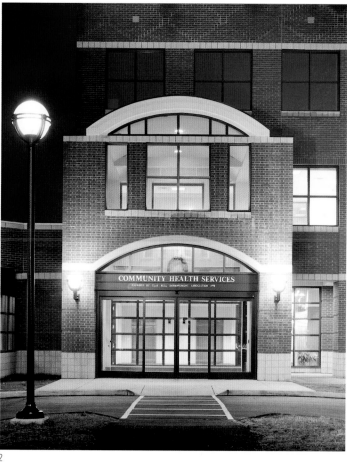

2

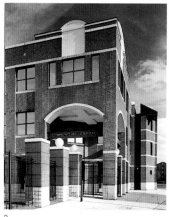

3

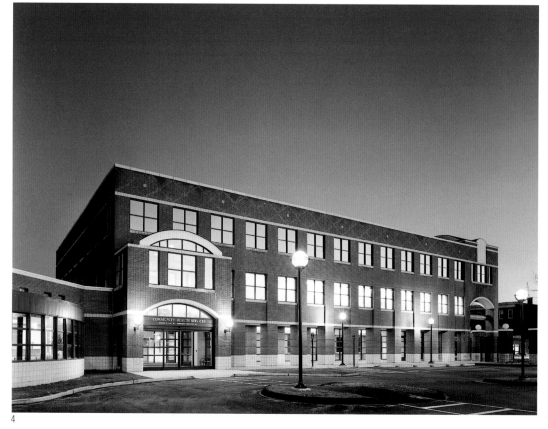

4

**Community Health Services
Connecticut, USA**
Du Bose Associates, Inc., Architects

1   Detail and texture relate to human scale
2   This two-storey entry lobby is
    neighborhood beacon
3   Articulated pavilion announces main
    entrance at street
4   Warm materials and large windows
    deinstitutionalize healthcare

Photo credit: Robert Benson Photography

**Blood Bank and Laboratories
Parramatta, NSW, Australia**
Ancher Mortlock and Woolley

5   Entrance at night
6   Entrance from small square
7   Café for donors

Photo credit: Eric Sierins

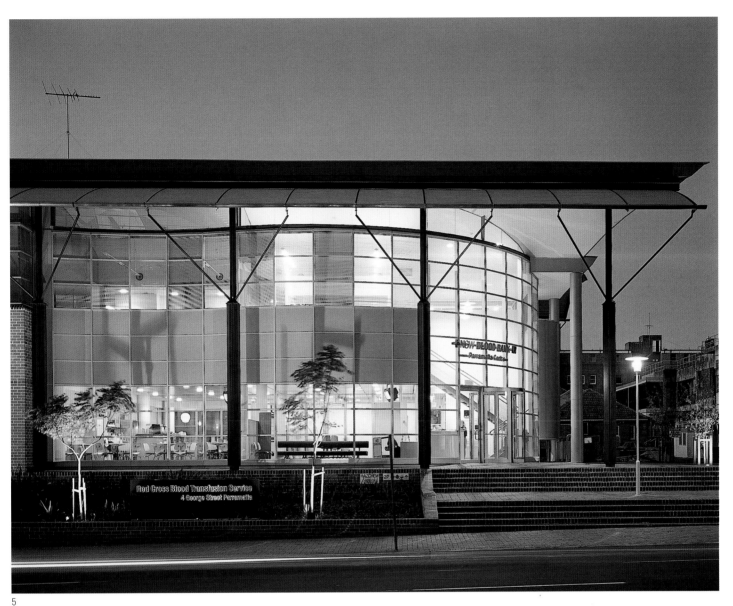

5

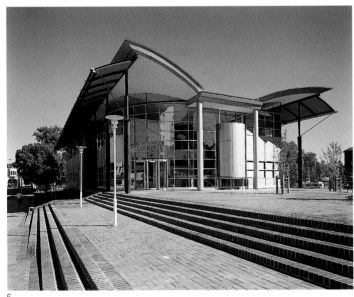

6

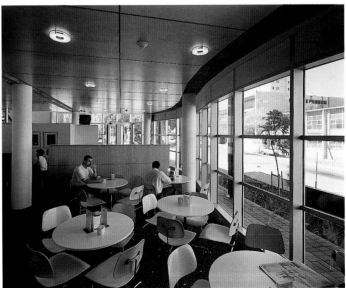

7

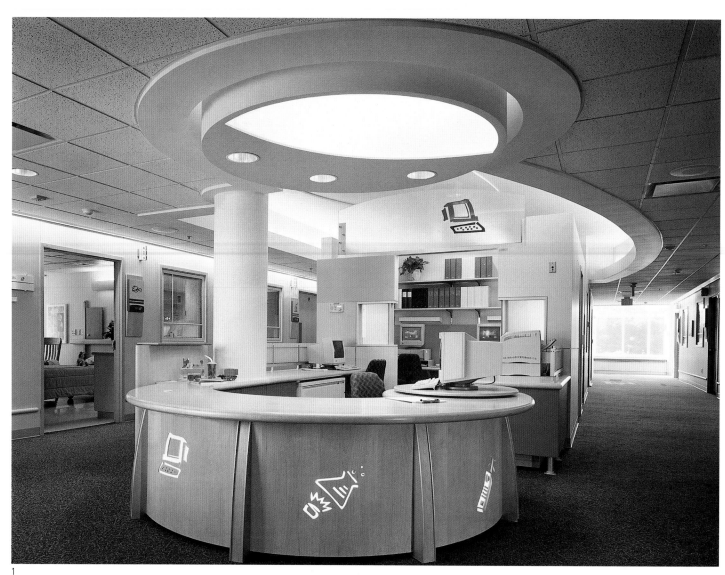

1

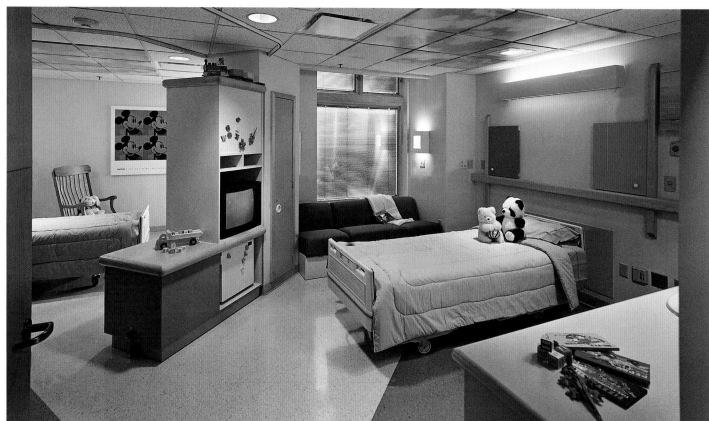

2

**Rainbow Babies and Children's Hospital
Cleveland, Ohio, USA**
NBBJ

1   186-bed tower addition complements
    existing facility
2   Patient rooms are designed to reflect
    familiar comfortable settings
Photo credit: Timothy Hursley

**Carl J. Shapiro Clinical Center
Massachusetts, USA**
Rothman Partners

3   Typical upper floor patient reception/
    waiting area
4   Atrium view towards family lounge
5   View from family lounge to entrance
6   View of atrium family lounge from fifth
    floor corridor
Photo credit: Steve Rosenthal

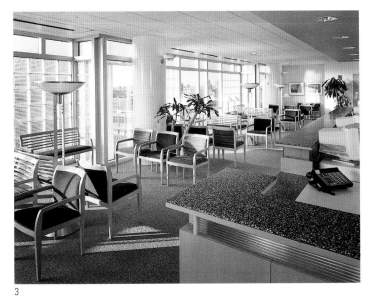

3

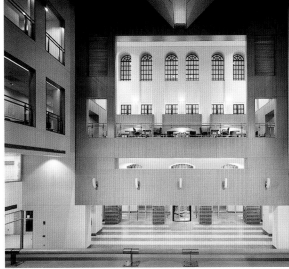

4

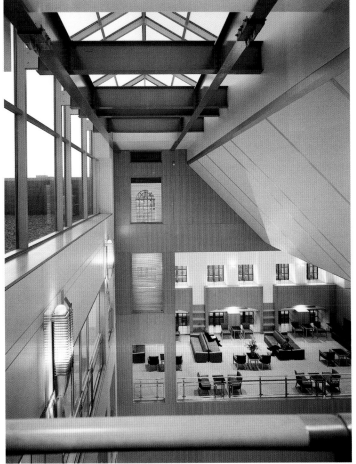

5

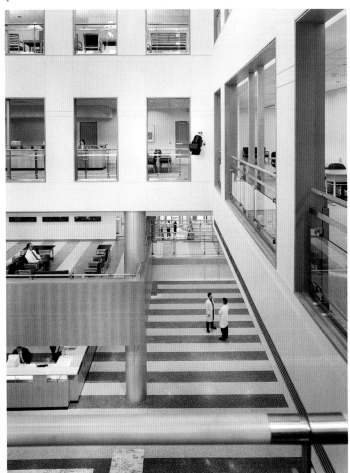

6

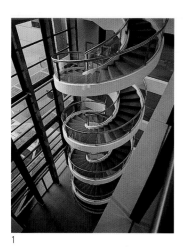

1

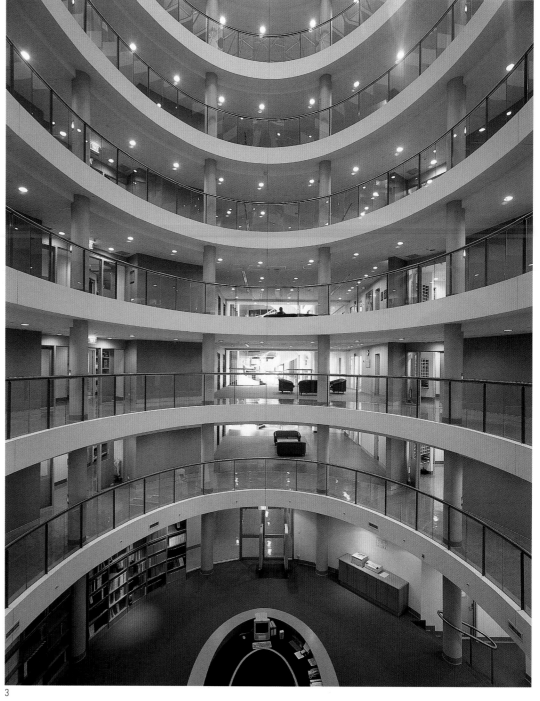

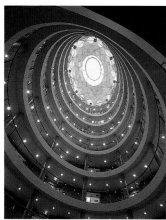

2

3

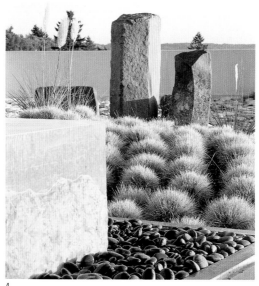

4

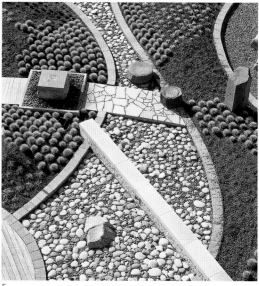

5

**Garvan Institute of Medical Research
Darlinghurst, NSW, Australia**
Ancher Mortlock and Woolley

1   Spiral stair in foyer area
2   Elevated view of atrium
3   Atrium with entrance gallery beyond
Photo credit: Eric Sierins

**Harrison Memorial Hospital
Bremerton, Washington, USA**
NBBJ

4   Rooftop landscaping and garden reflect
     regional settings
5   Aerial view of rooftop garden
6   Exterior of NBBJ's surgery addition
Photo credits: Paul Warchol (4); Steve Keating
(5&6)

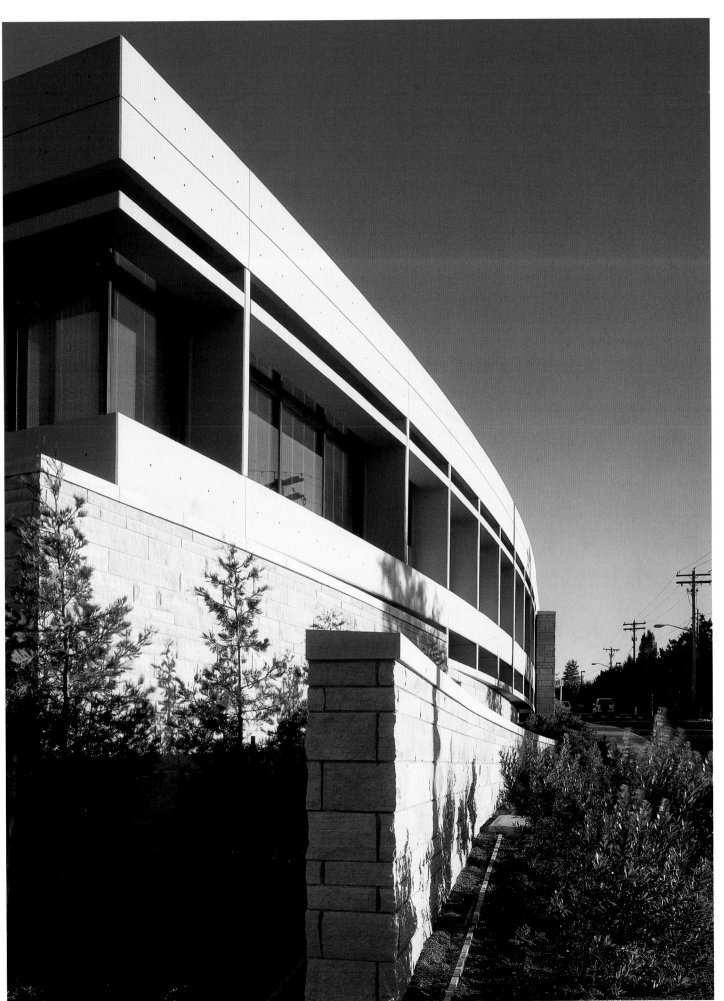

Phoebe Northwest, Phoebe Putney
Memorial Hospital
Albany, Georgia, USA
TRO/The Ritchie Organization

1   Exercise equipment in rehabilitation
    room
2   Large interior physical medicine space
    was subdivided to create privacy zones
3   Mezzanine level added to accommodate
    a 1/15-mile walking track
Photo credit: George Cott

Sutter Santa Cruz Maternity
and Surgical Center
Santa Cruz, California, USA
Kaplan McLaughlin Diaz in association
with Silva Strong Architects

4   Exterior view of patient room windows
    and recessed balconies
5   French doors of LDRP suites open onto
    exterior balconies
Photo credit: Erich Anset Koyama

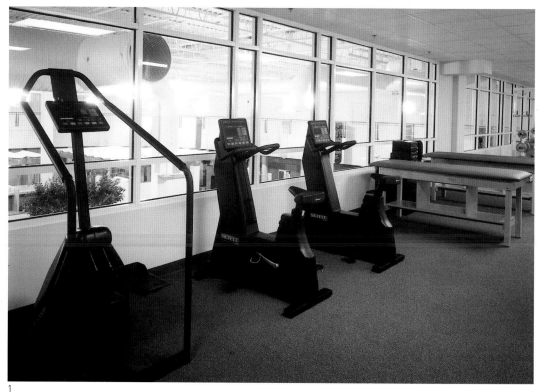

1

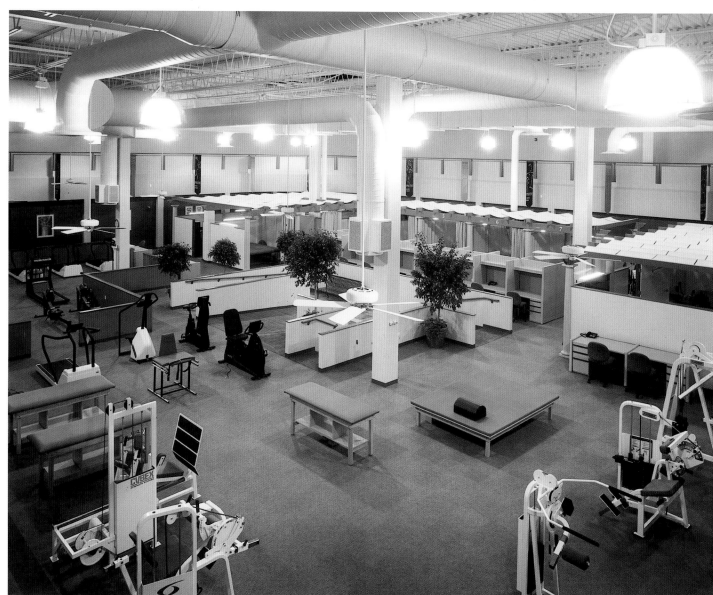

2

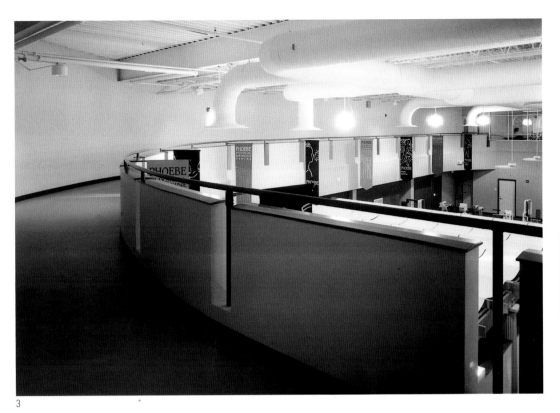

3

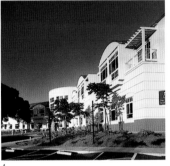

4

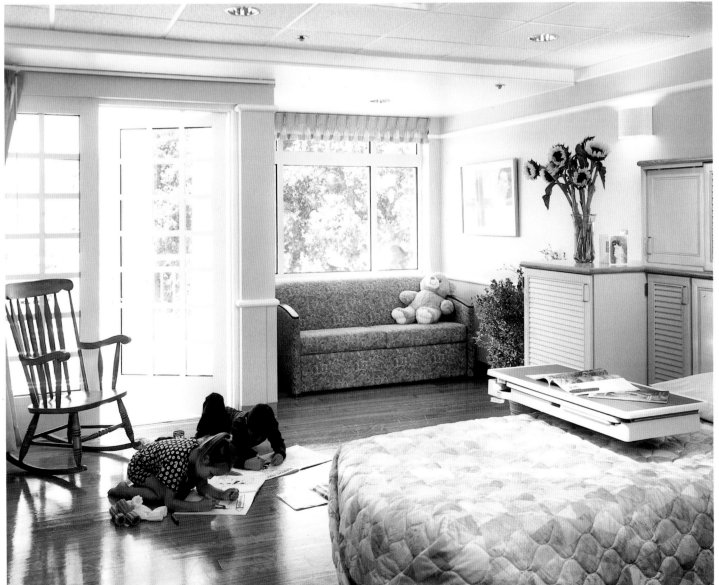

5

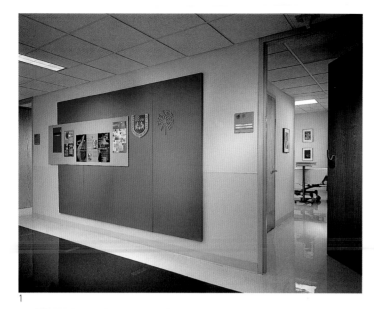

1

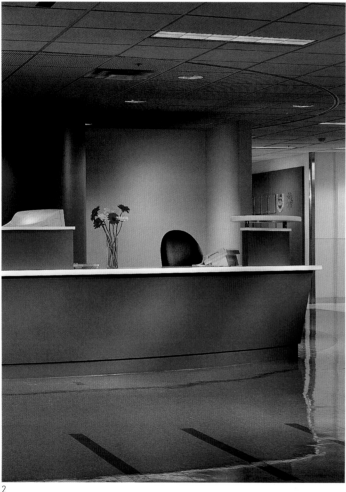

2

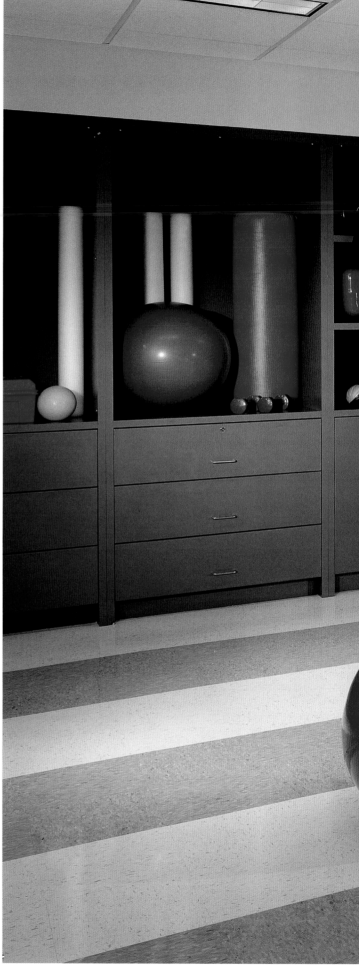

Loyola University Medical Center
Maywood, Illinois, USA
RTKL Associates Inc.

1   Rehabilitation Center's interior corridor
2   Rehabilitation reception area
3   Rehabilitation room

Photo credit: Craig Dugan/Hedrich-Blessing

3

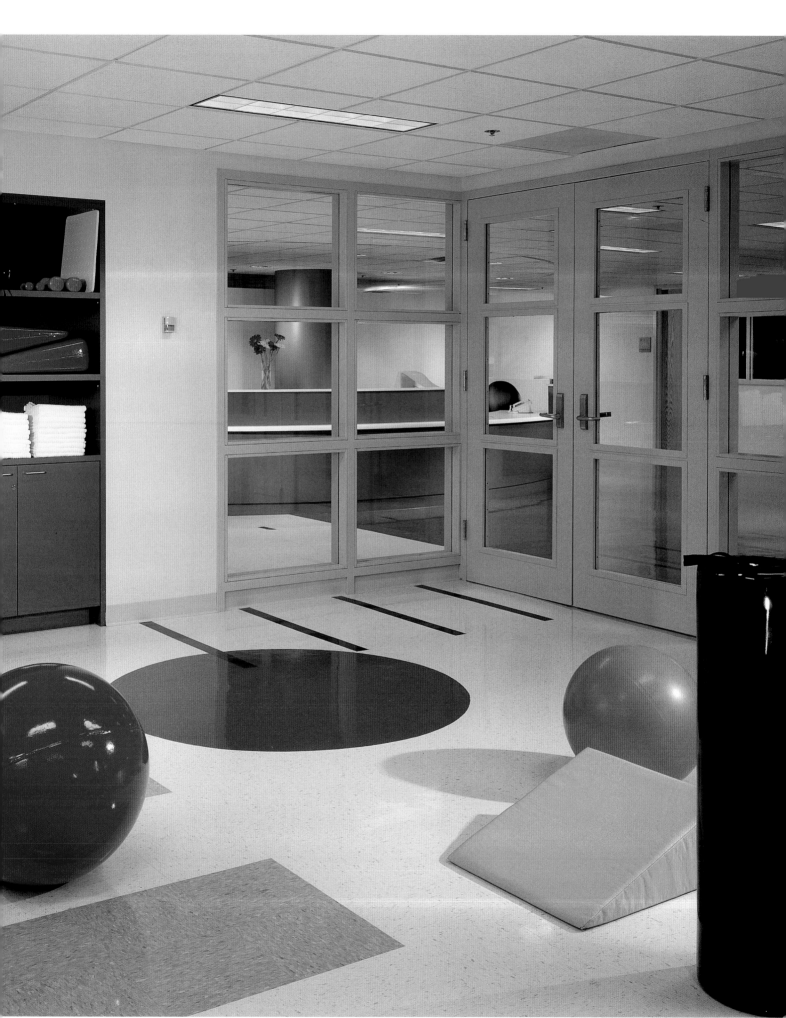

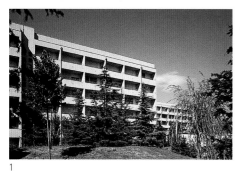

1

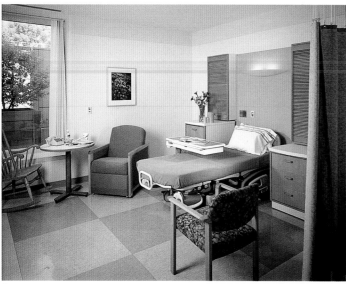

2

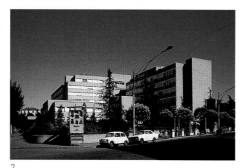

3

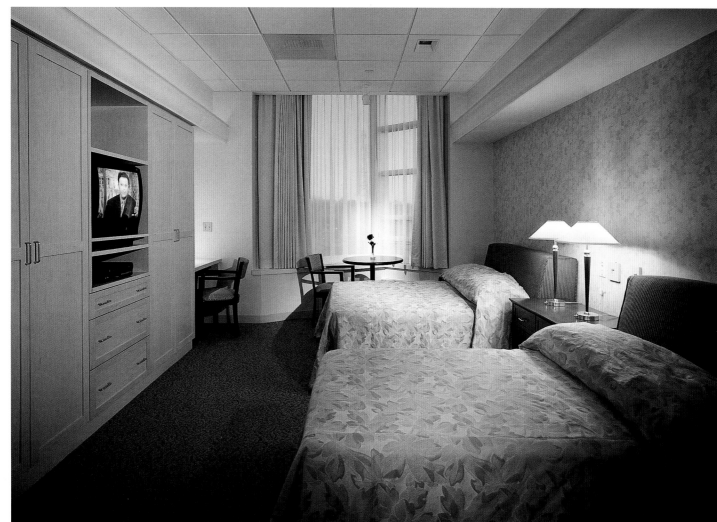

4

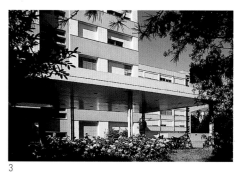

5

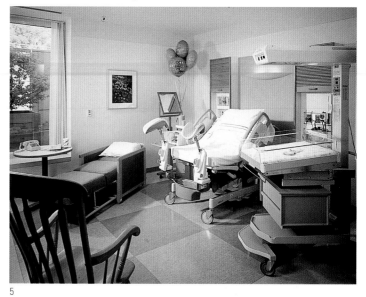

6

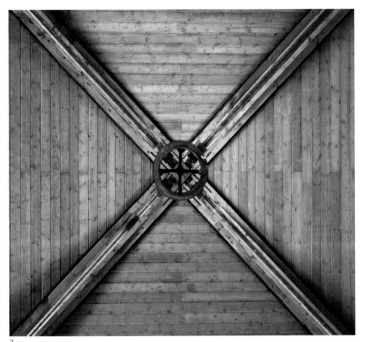

Ospedale Specializzato Marcello Malpighi
Bologna, Italy
Enzo Zacchiroli Architetto

1–3   General view of hospital exterior
Photo credit: courtesy of Enzo Zacchiroli Architetto

Kaiser Vallejo Hospital
Vallejo, California, USA
Skidmore, Owings & Merrill LLP

4   LDR, Labour arrangement
5   LDR, Delivery arrangement
Photo credit: courtesy of Skidmore, Owings & Merrill LLP

University of Nebraska,
Lied Transplant Center
Omaha, Nebraska, USA
Hellmuth, Obata + Kassabaum, Inc.
in association with Leo A Daly

6   View of Cooperative Care Room
Photo credit: Paul Brokering

Rehabilitation Center
Trassenheide, Usedom, Germany
gmp–von Gerkan Marg & Partner

7   Tower ceiling
8   Tower exterior
9   Pitched zinc roofs create hospital vernacular
Photo credit: Klaus Frahm

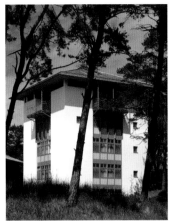

7

8

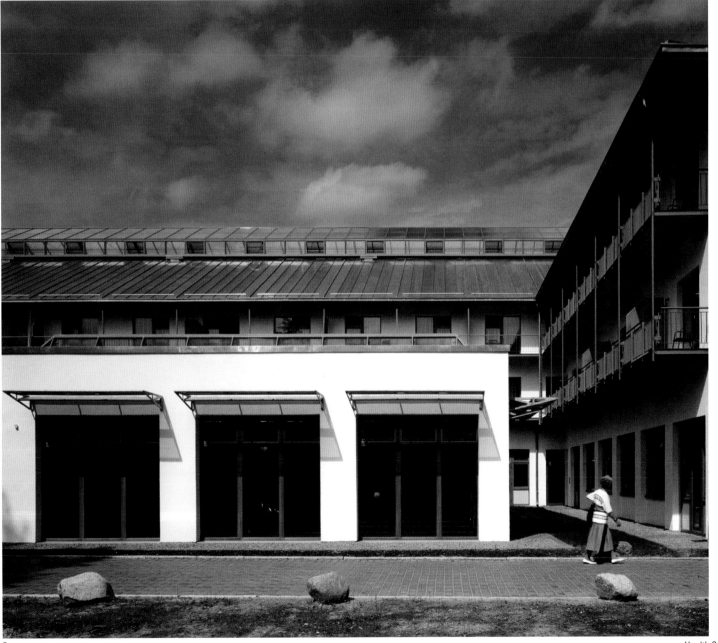

9

Harrison Memorial Hospital
Bremerton, Washington, USA
NBBJ

1   Operating room
2   Main operating room corridor
Photo credit: Steve Keating

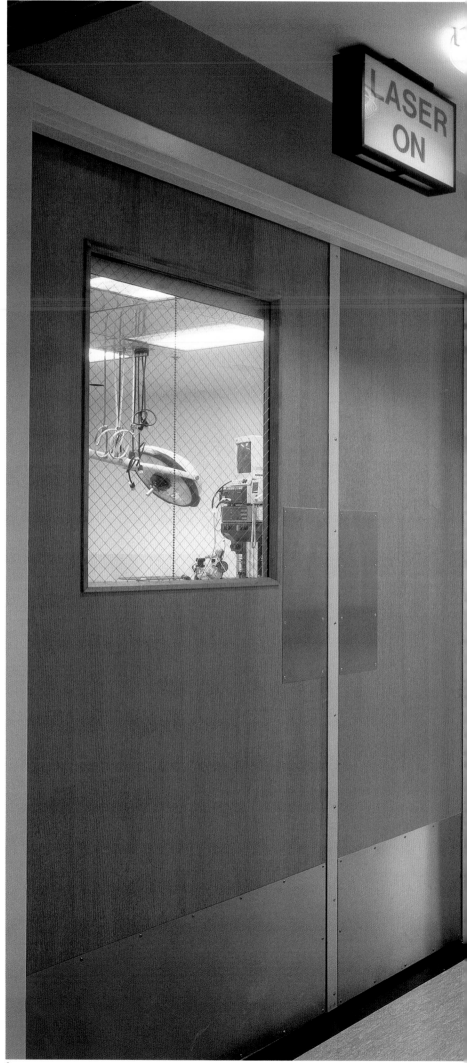

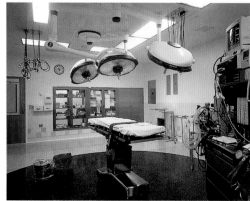

1

2

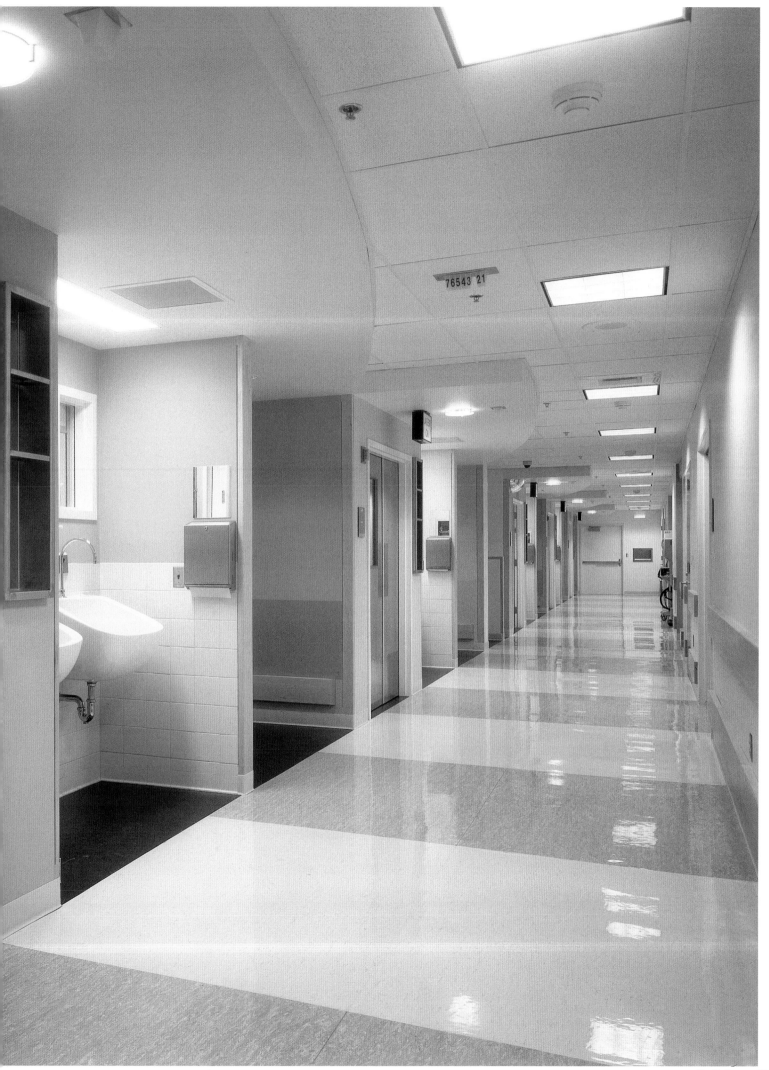

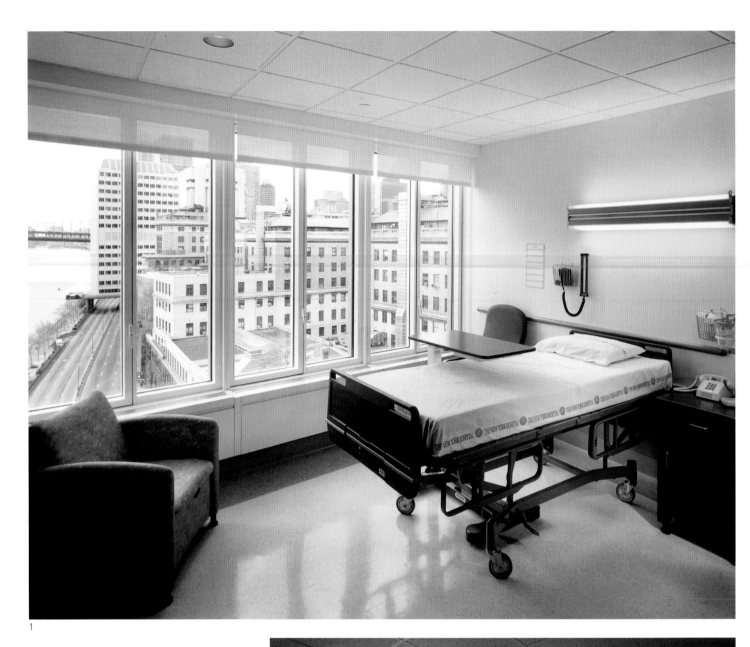

1

The New York Hospital
New York, USA
Hellmuth, Obata + Kassabaum, Inc.
1   Intensive Care Unit bed
2   Acute Care patient room
Photo credit: courtesy of Hellmuth, Obata + Kassabaum, Inc.

Salon de Provence Hospital
Salon de Provence, France
BDP Groupe 6
3   Main entrance hall
Photo credit: courtesy of BDP Groupe 6

Resurrection Medical Center
Chicago, Illinois, USA
Loebl Schlossman & Hackl
4   Paediatric Department's playroom
5   Life Center bedroom
Following pages:
     Life Center bedroom
Photo credit: Bruce VanInwegen

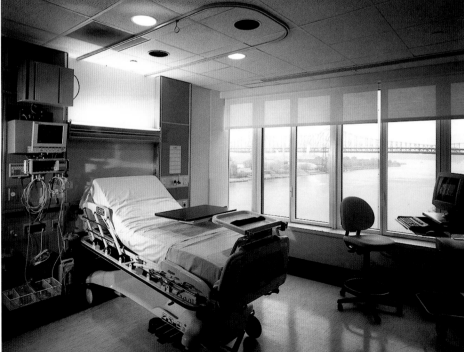

2

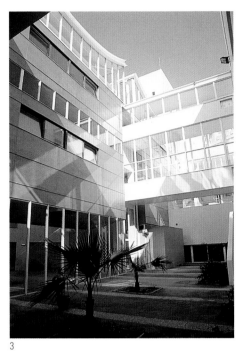

3

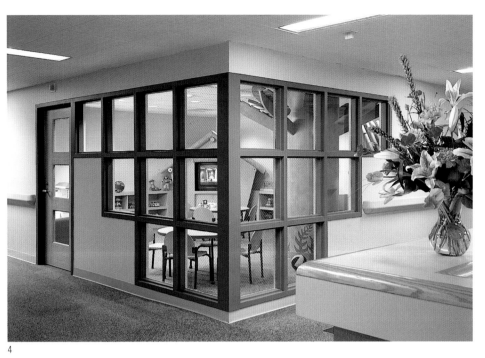

4

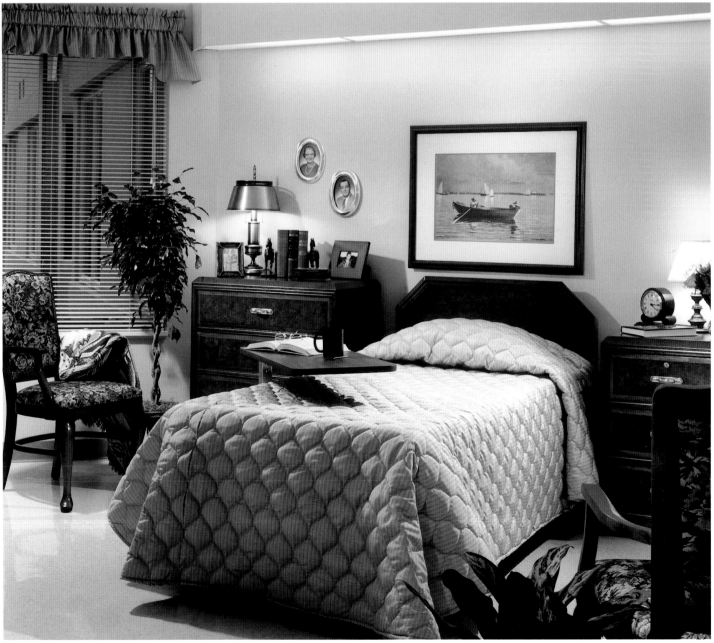

5

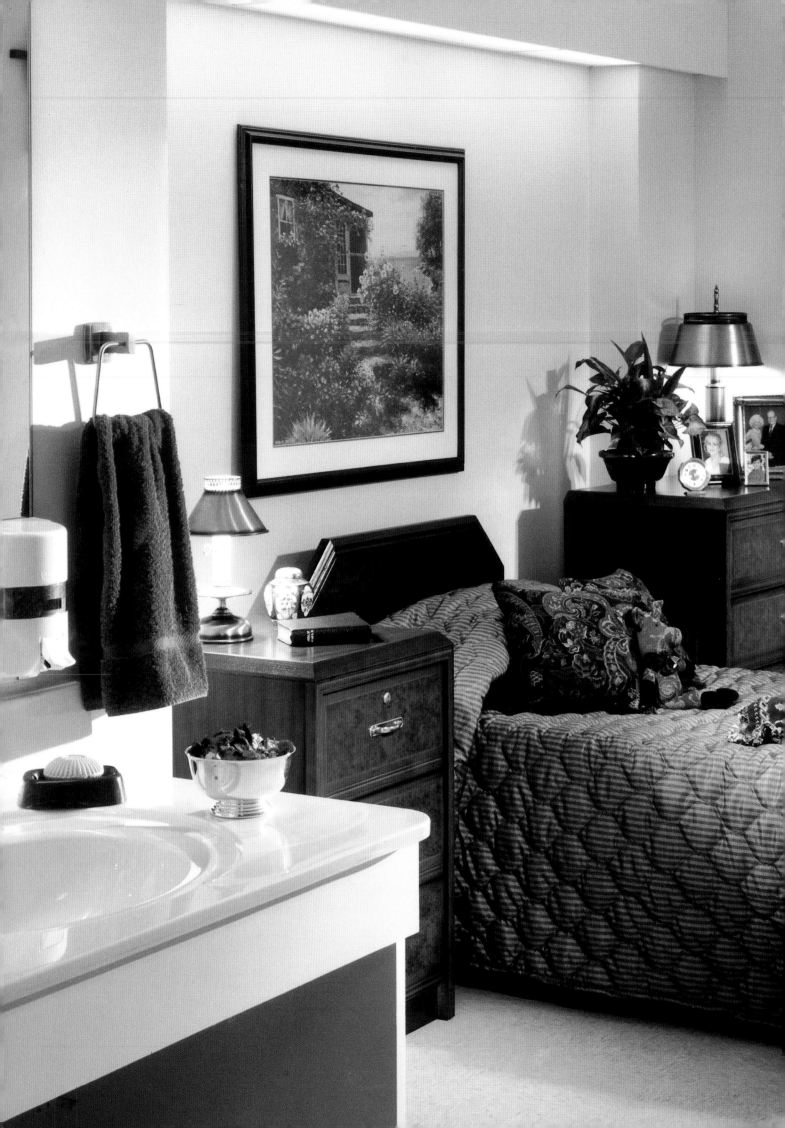

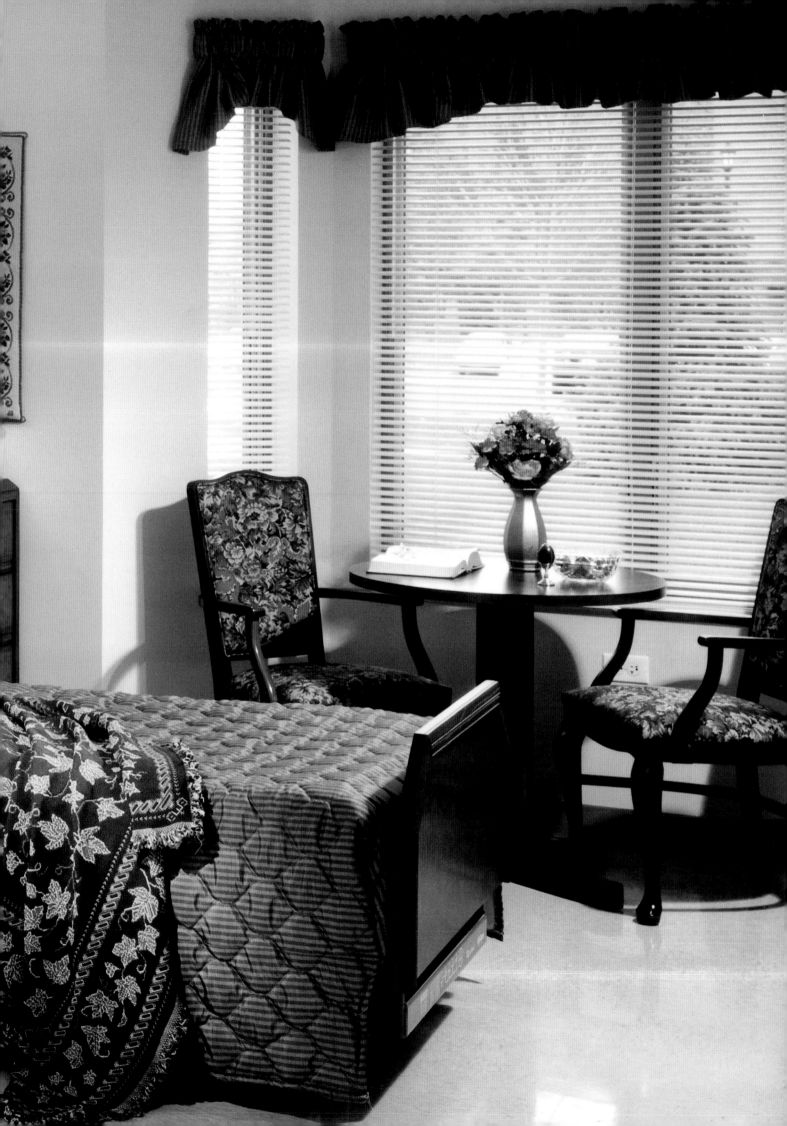

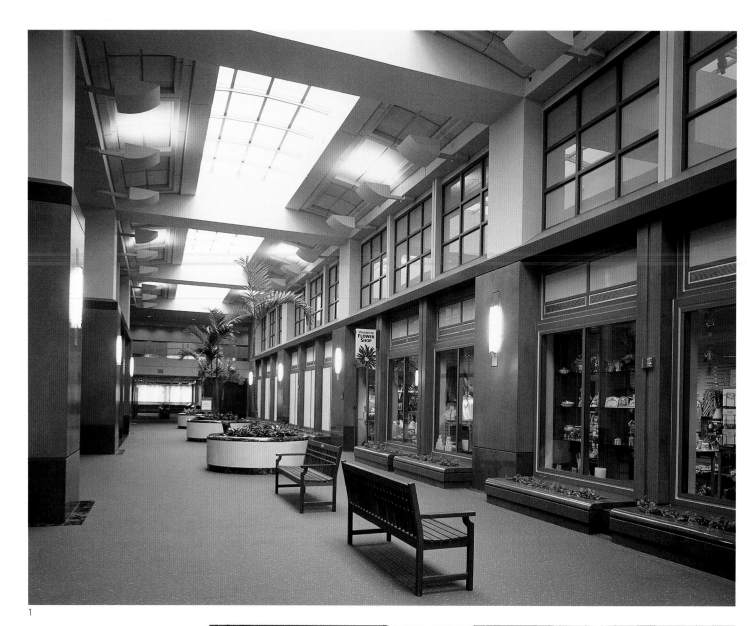

1

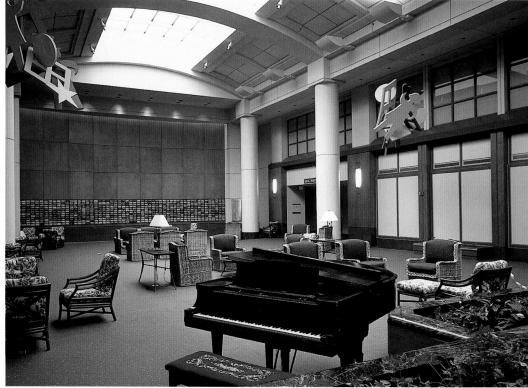

MD Anderson Cancer Center
Houston, Texas, USA
LAN/HKS Inc. Joint Venture

1&2   Waiting area
3   Public space called the Pedi-Dome
Photo credit: Rick Gardner

2

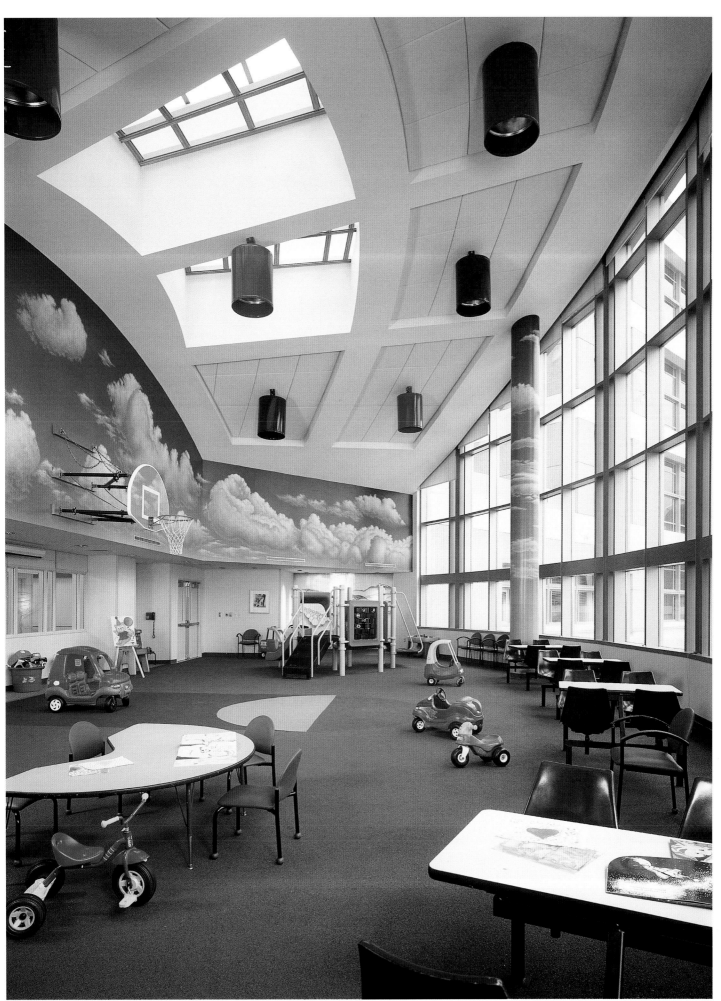

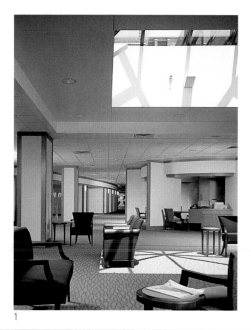

1

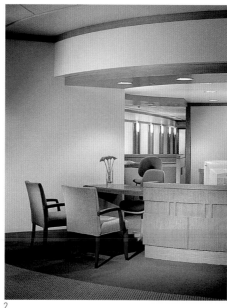

2

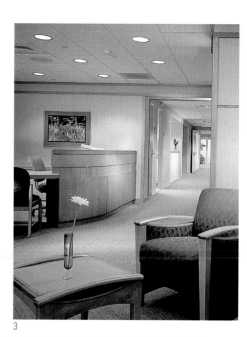

3

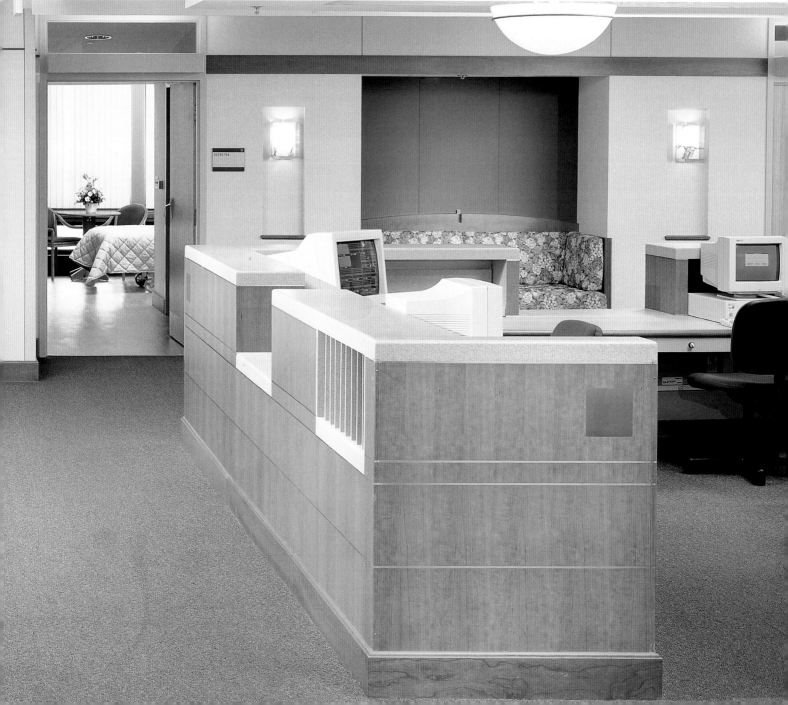

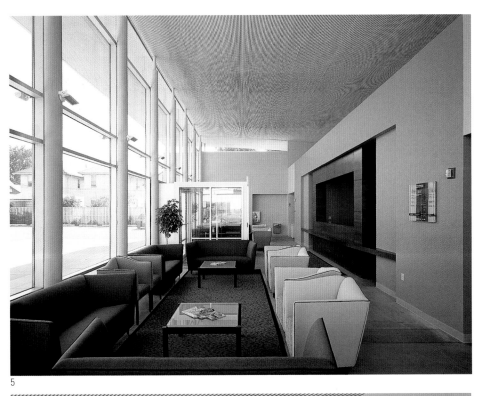

5

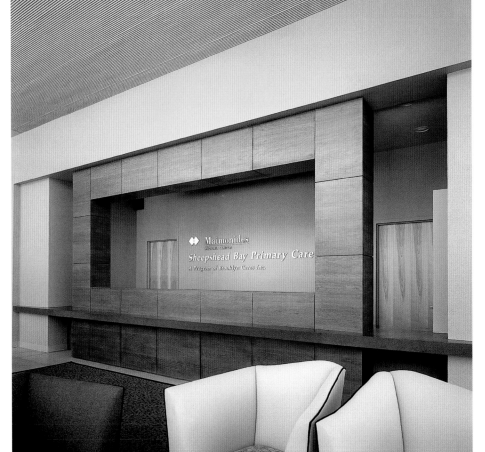

6

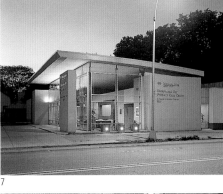

7

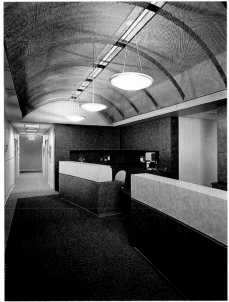

8

**St. Michael's Hospital
Stevens Point, Wisconsin, USA**
Flad & Associates
1   Skylight brings in daylight to warm and
    illuminate waiting area
2   Central registration hub greets
    ambulatory surgery patients
3   Rich wood and natural tones colour
    Cancer Center entrance
Photo credit: Christopher Barrett

**Anne Arundel Medical Center, Rebecca
M. Clatanoff Women's Hospital
Maryland, USA**
RTKL Associates Inc.
Opposite bottom:
    Nurses' station
Photo credit: Max MacKenzie

**Maimonides Medical Center, Sheepshead
Bay Primary Care Center
Brooklyn, New York, USA**
Lee Harris Pomeroy Associates/Architects
5   Glass wall along edge of waiting room
6   Main reception desk
7   Evening illumination of main waiting area
8   Nurses' station
Following pages:
    Illuminated interior provides welcoming
    reception for visitors
Photo credit: Christopher Lovi

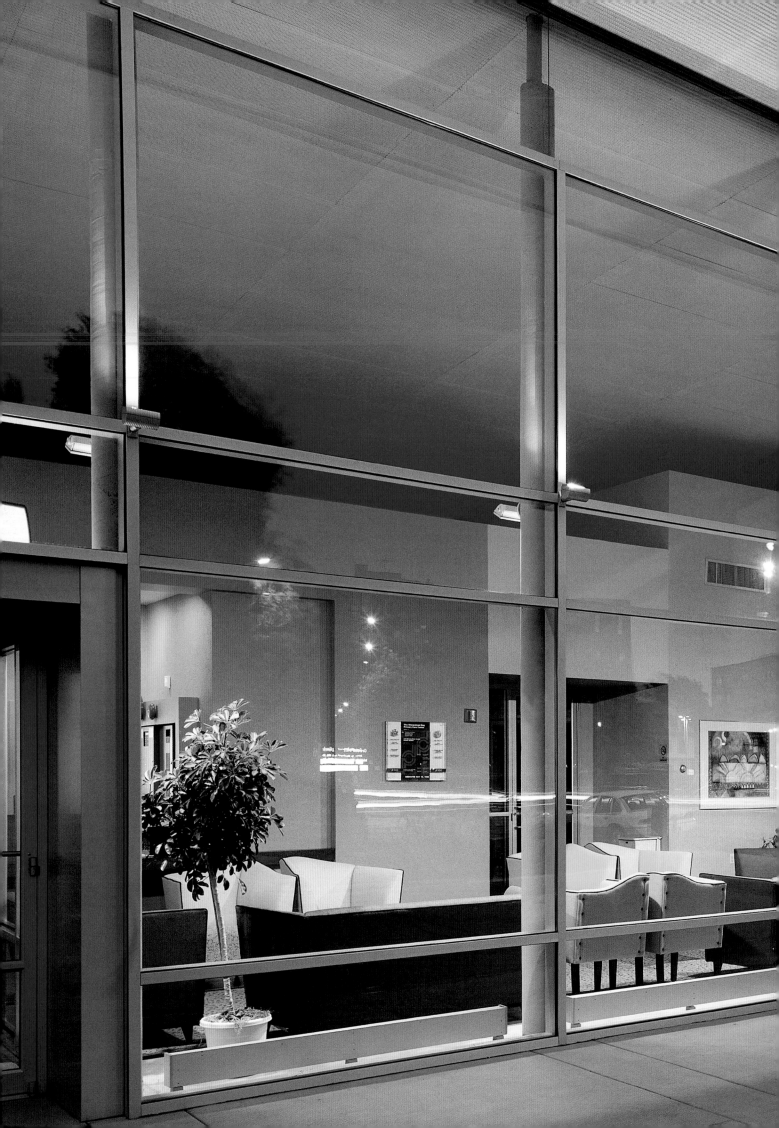

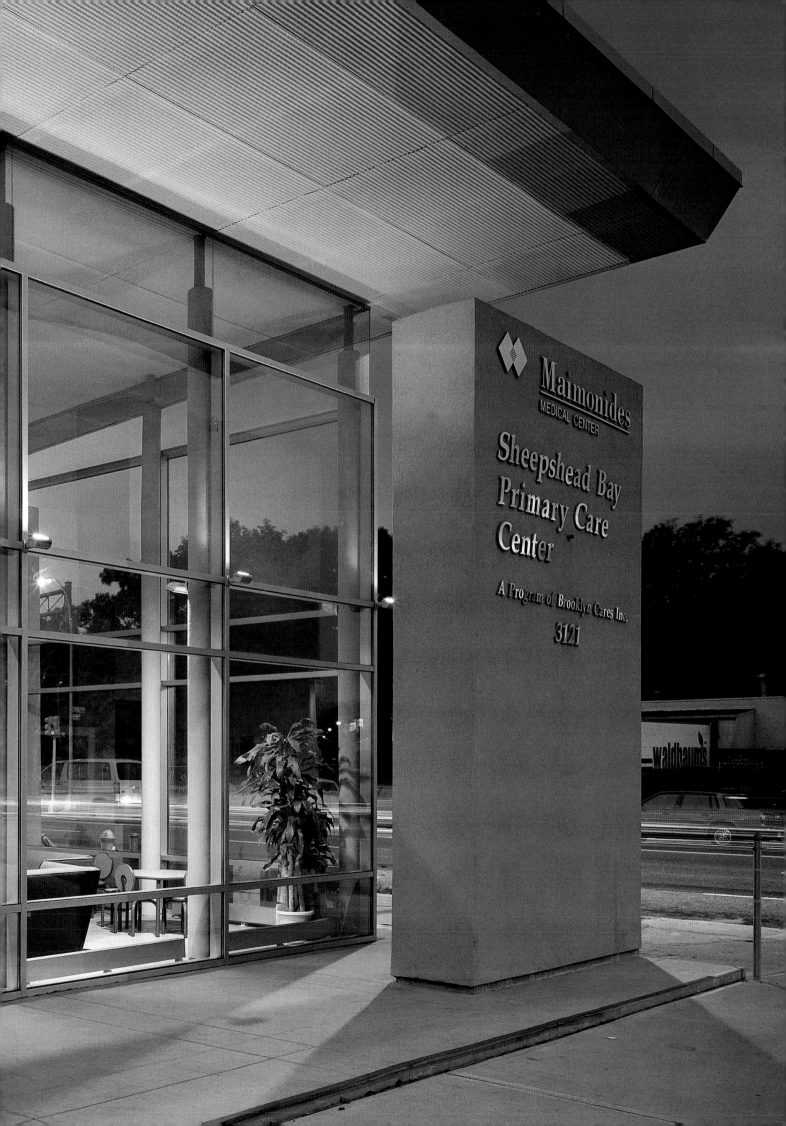

**Kauniala Disabled War Veteran's Hospital
Kauniala, Finland**
Paatela & Paatela Architects

1 Kitchen
2 Dining
Photo credit: Timo Kauppila

**Rehabilitation Institute of
Chicago Northshore
Northbrook, Illinois, USA**
Loebl Schlossman & Hackl

3 Day therapy
4 Rehabilitation
Photo credit: Bruce VanInwegen

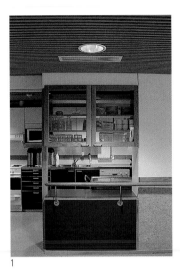

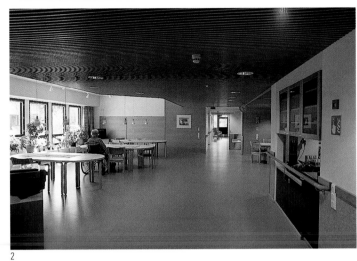

1

2

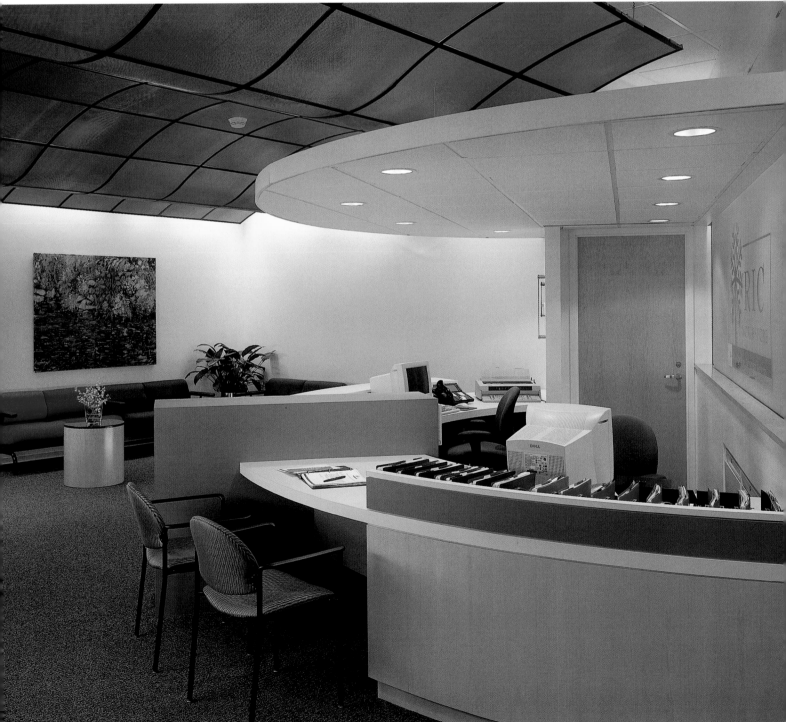

3

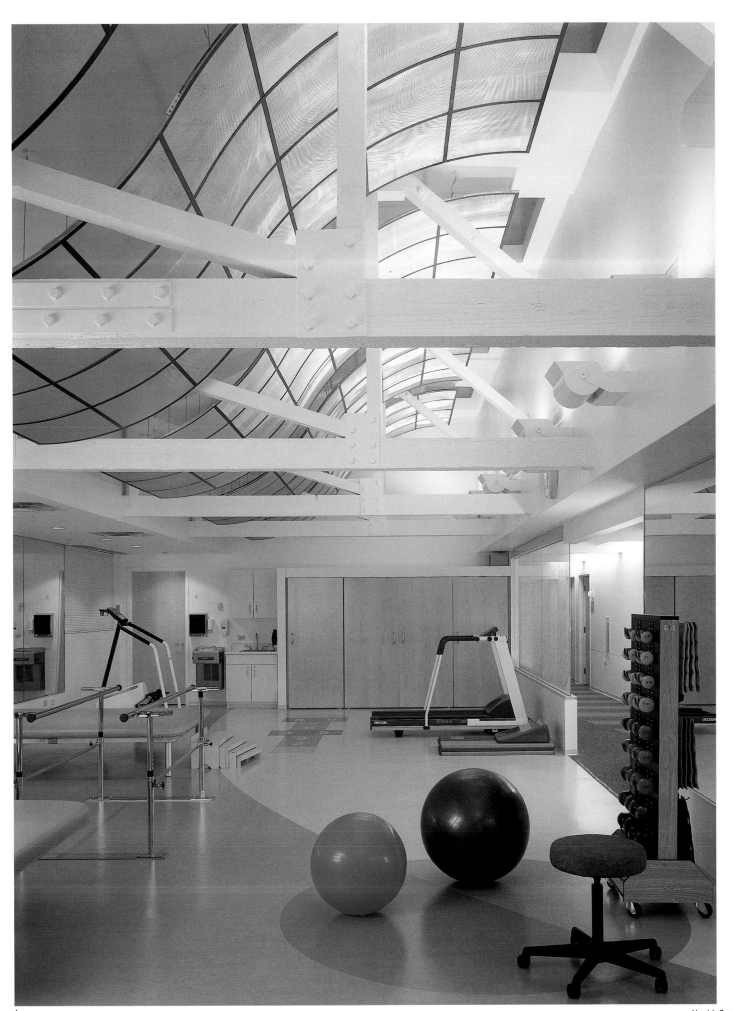

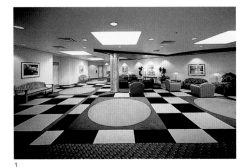

1

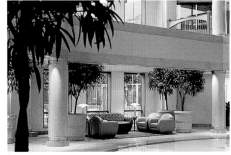

2

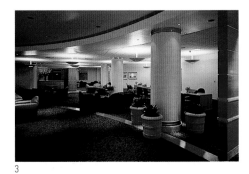

3

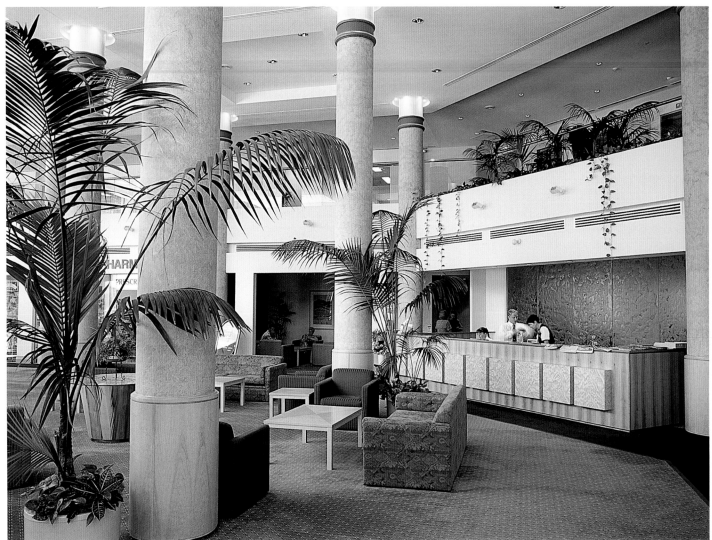

4

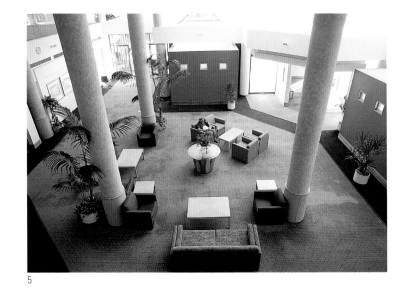

5

All Saints Episcopal Hospital
Fort Worth, Texas, USA
HKS Inc.

1　Bold colours and geometric shapes create
　　an energetic environment
2　Atrium and lobby depict familiar aspects of
　　city and state
3　Waiting area

Photo credit: Wes Thompson

John Flynn Medical Centre
Tugun, Queensland, Australia
Woods Bagot

4　Main entrance
5　Atrium
6&9　Waiting area
7　Corridor view
8　Staff base
10　Consulting room

Photo credit: courtesy of Woods Bagot

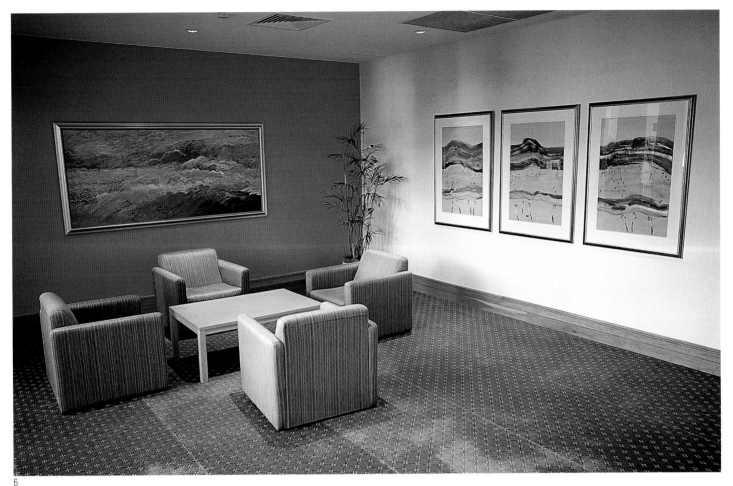

6

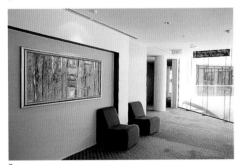

7

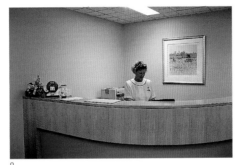

8

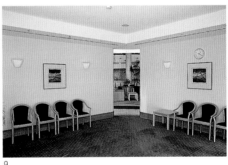

9

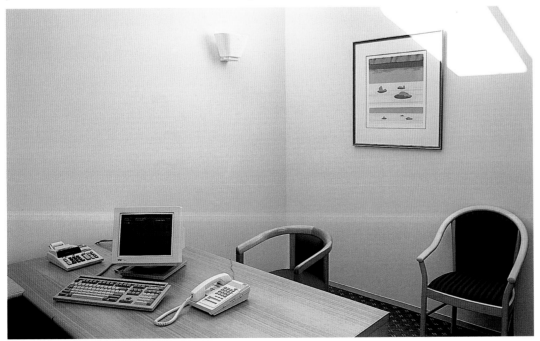

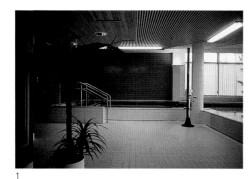

1

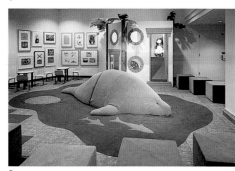

2

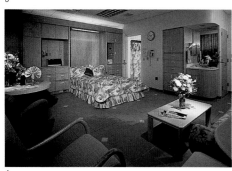

3

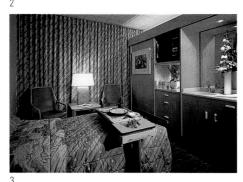

4

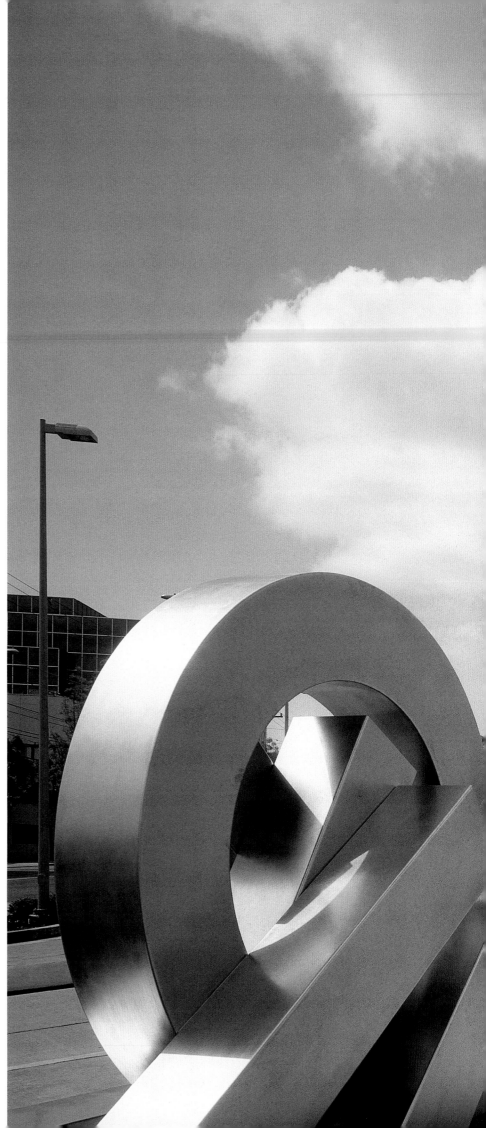

Vaasa Central Hospital
Vaasa, Finland
Paatela & Paatela Architects
1   Rehabilitation swimming pool
Photo credit: courtesy of Paatela & Paatela Architects

HealthPark Medical Center
Fort Myers, Florida, USA
HKS Inc.
2   Paediatric play area
3   Patient room at night
4   LDPR room 'birthday suite'
Photo credit: Rick Grumbaum

Swedish Medical Center
Seattle, Washington, USA
NBBJ
Opposite:
    Main entrance to new southeast wing addition
Photo credit: Assassi Productions

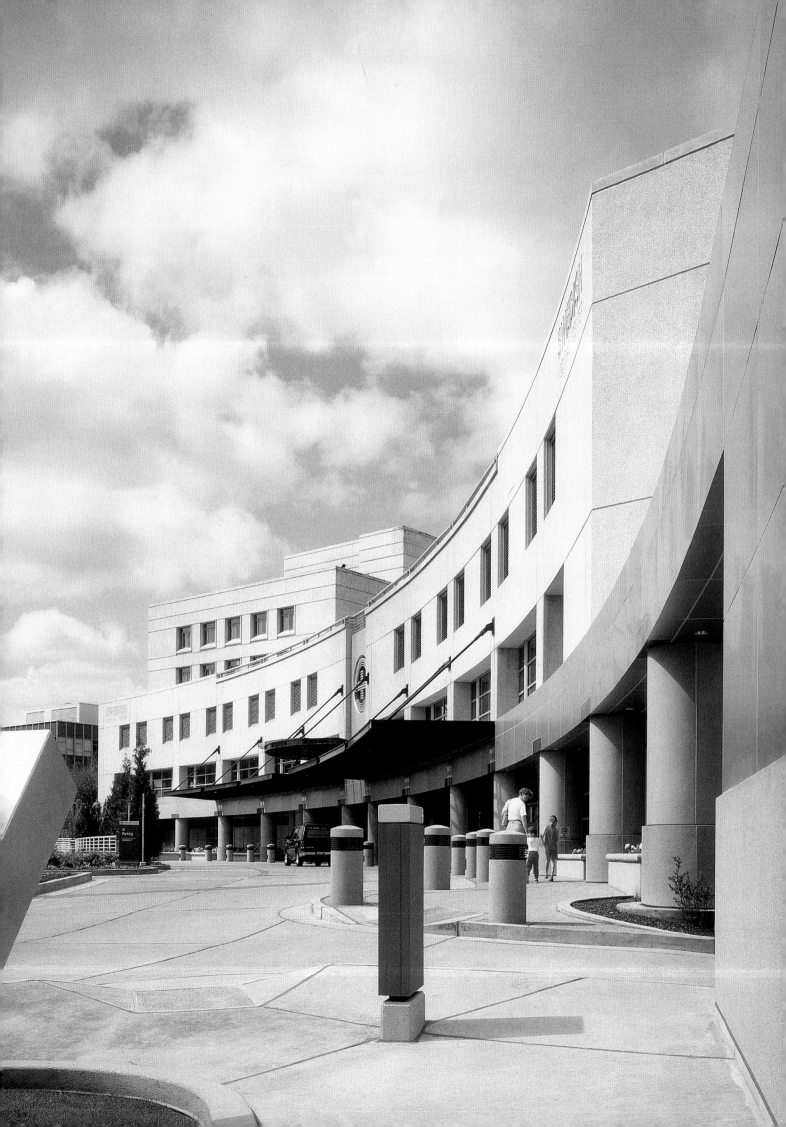

Barry Medical Park
Kansas City, Missouri, USA
WRS Architects Inc.

1 Four-storey medical office building with enclosed connection to adjacent hospital
2 East façade of medical office building
3 Multi-media Conference Center for public and professional community

Photo credit: Mike Sinclair Photography

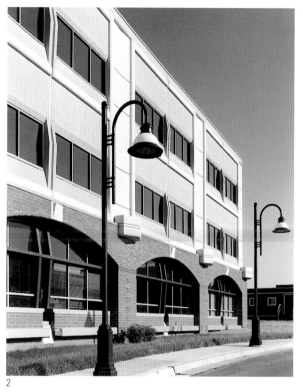

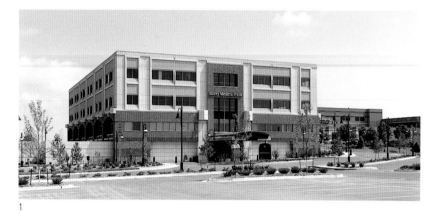

1

2

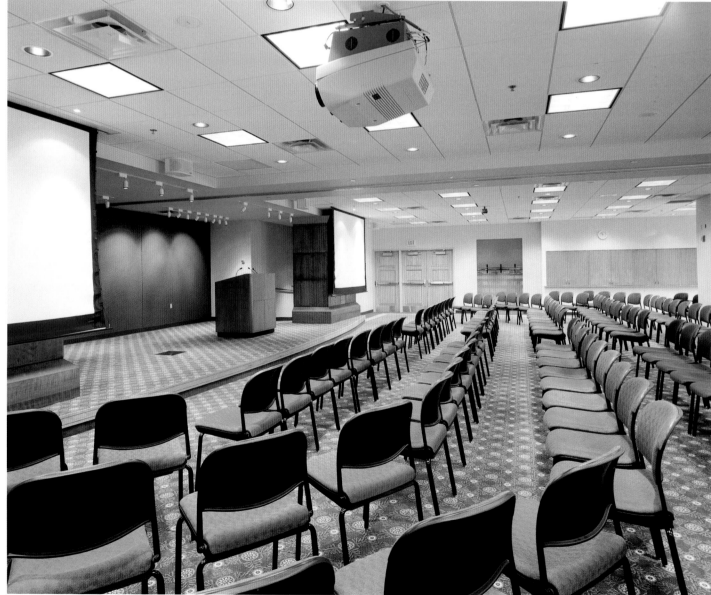

3

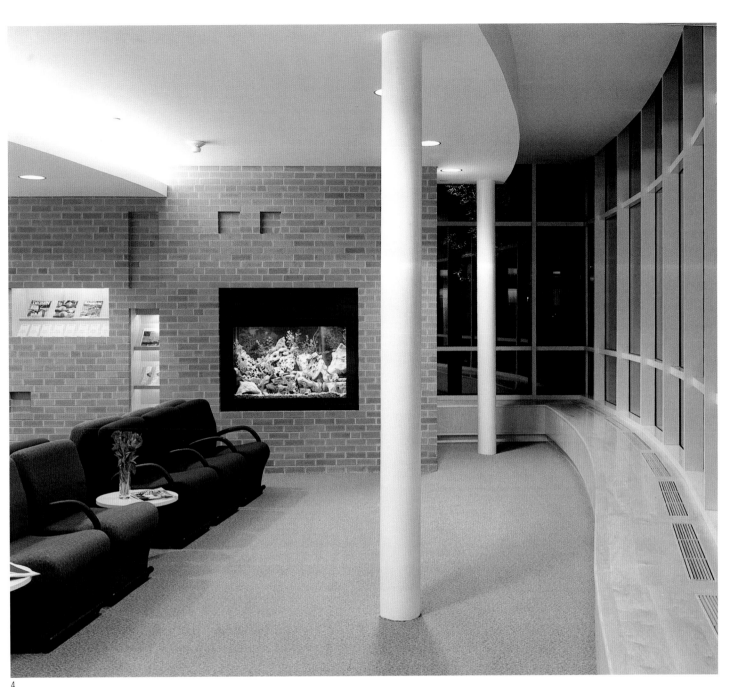

4

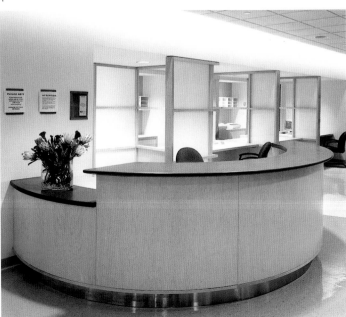

5

St. Mary's Health Center
Missouri, USA
Mackey Mitchell Associates

4 Waiting area
5 Triage and three registration niches
  provide fast service and improved privacy
Photo credit: courtesy of Mackey Mitchell
Associates

Pali Moni Hospital
Aiea, Hawaii
Media Five Limited

Following pages:
  Waiting area
Photo credit: Ron Starr

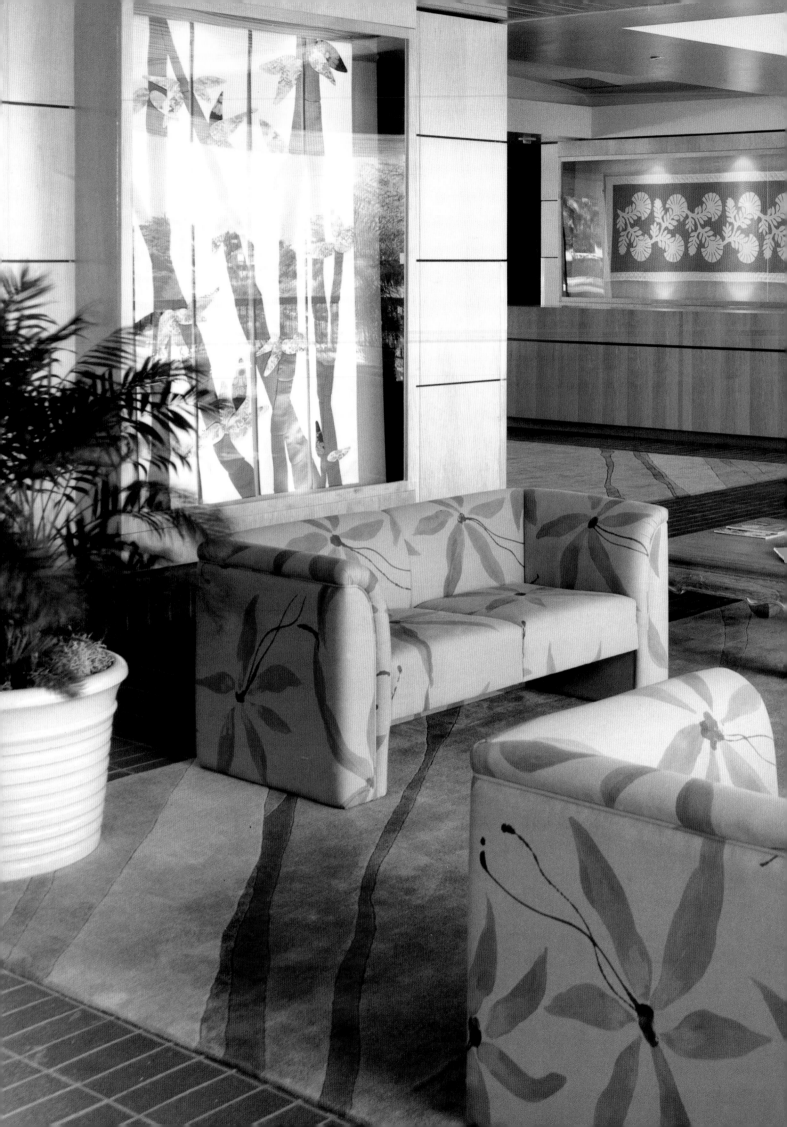

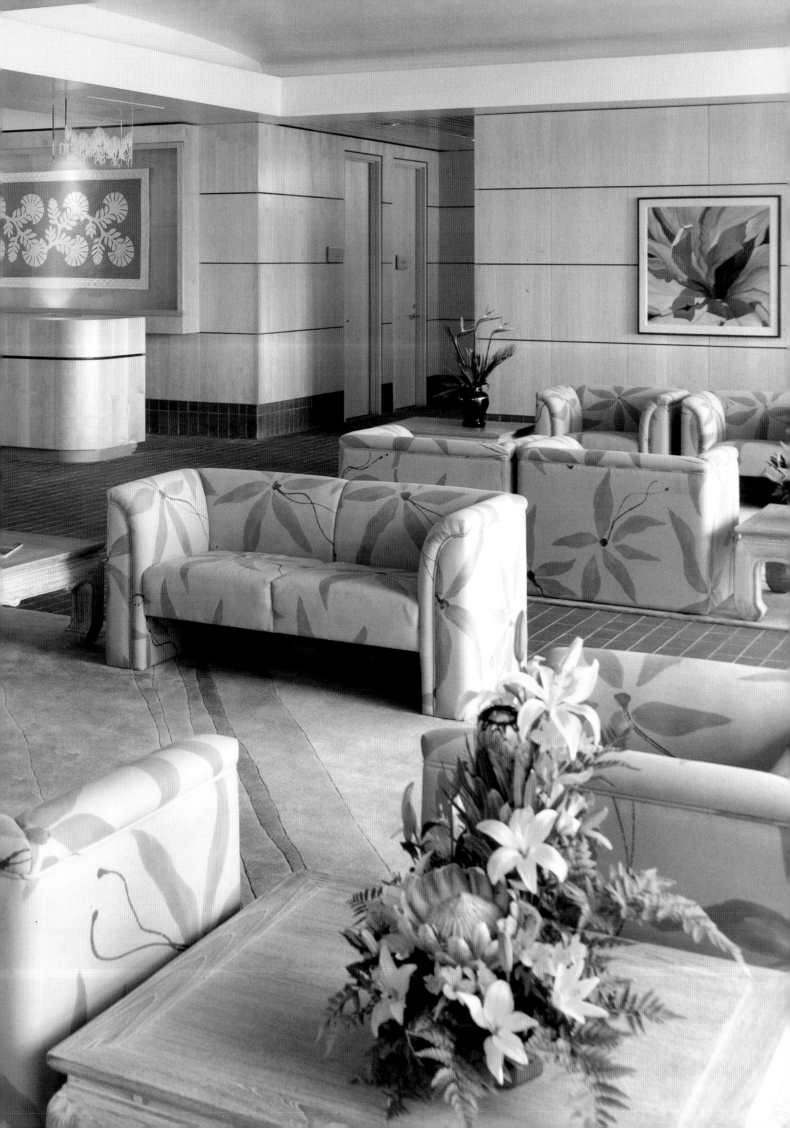

Montreuil sur Mer Hospital
Montreuil, France
BDP Groupe 6

1   Exterior of hospital building
Photo credit: courtesy of BDP Groupe 6

Health Central
Ocoee, Florida, USA
HKS Inc.

2   Typical patient room with four square
    windows
Photo credit: Rick Grumbaum & Michael Lowry

Pomona Valley Hospital Medical Center
Pomona, California, USA
NBBJ

3   Interior of wards
Photo credit: courtesy of NBBJ

Helsinki University Central Hospital for
Skin and Allergic Diseases
Helskini, Finland
Paatela & Paatela Architects

4   South elevation
5   Aerial view
Photo credits: Timo Kauppila (4); Gero Mylius (5)

Connecticut Children's Hospital
Hartford, Connecticut, USA
HKS Inc.

6   Reception area
7   Entry detail
8   Elevator lobby area
Photo credit: Robert Benson Photography

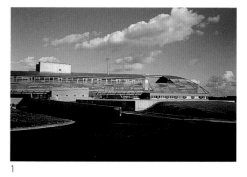

1

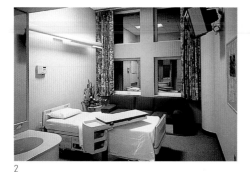

2

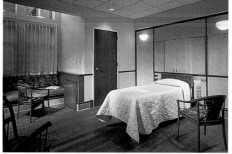

3

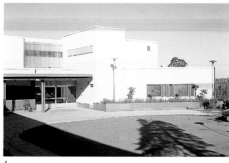

4

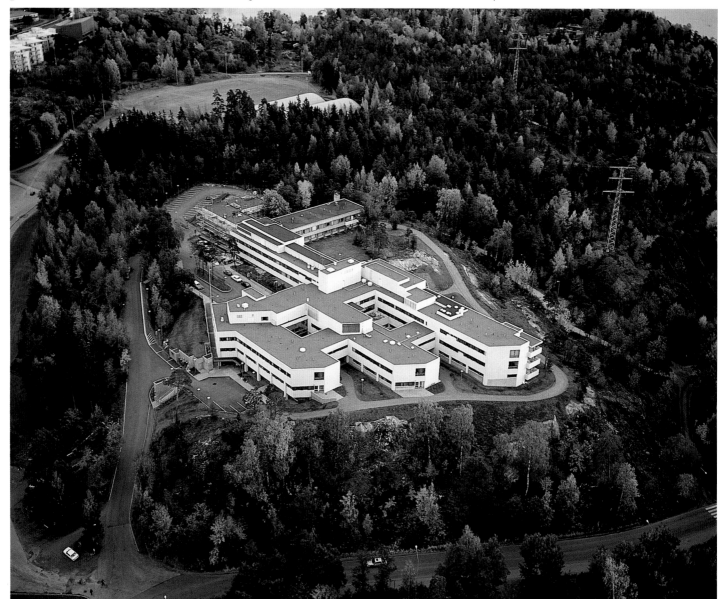

5

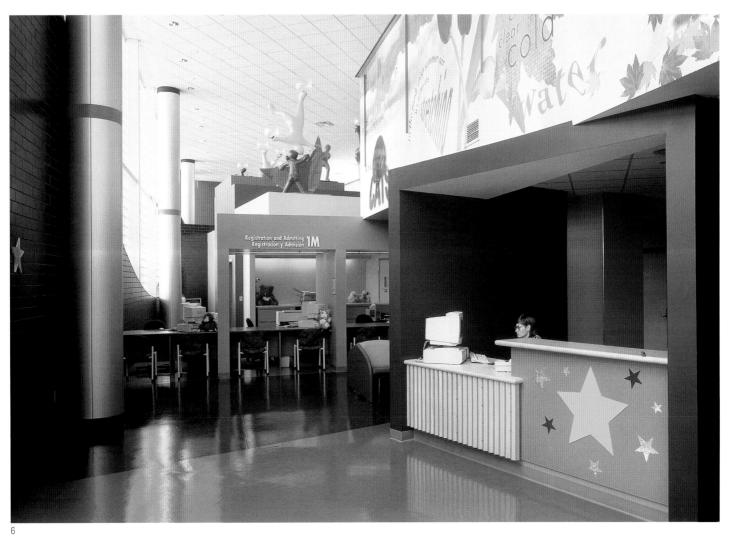

6

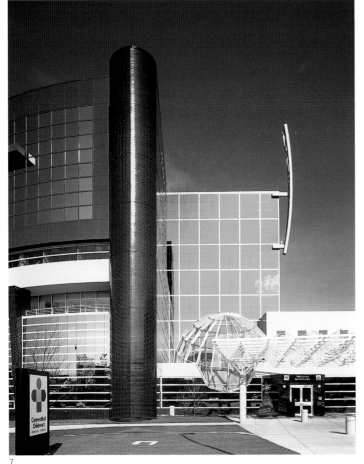

7

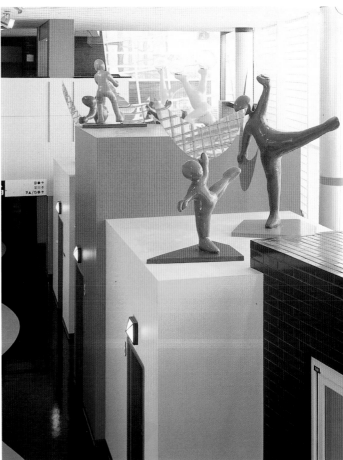

8

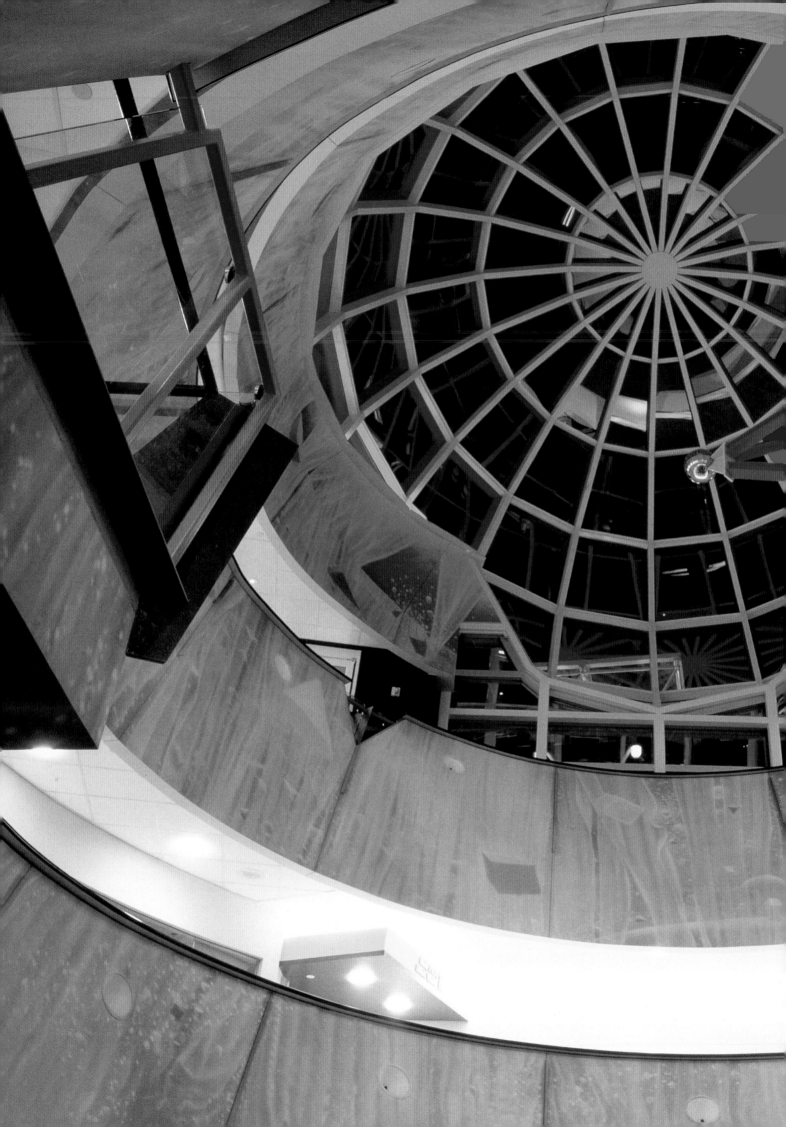

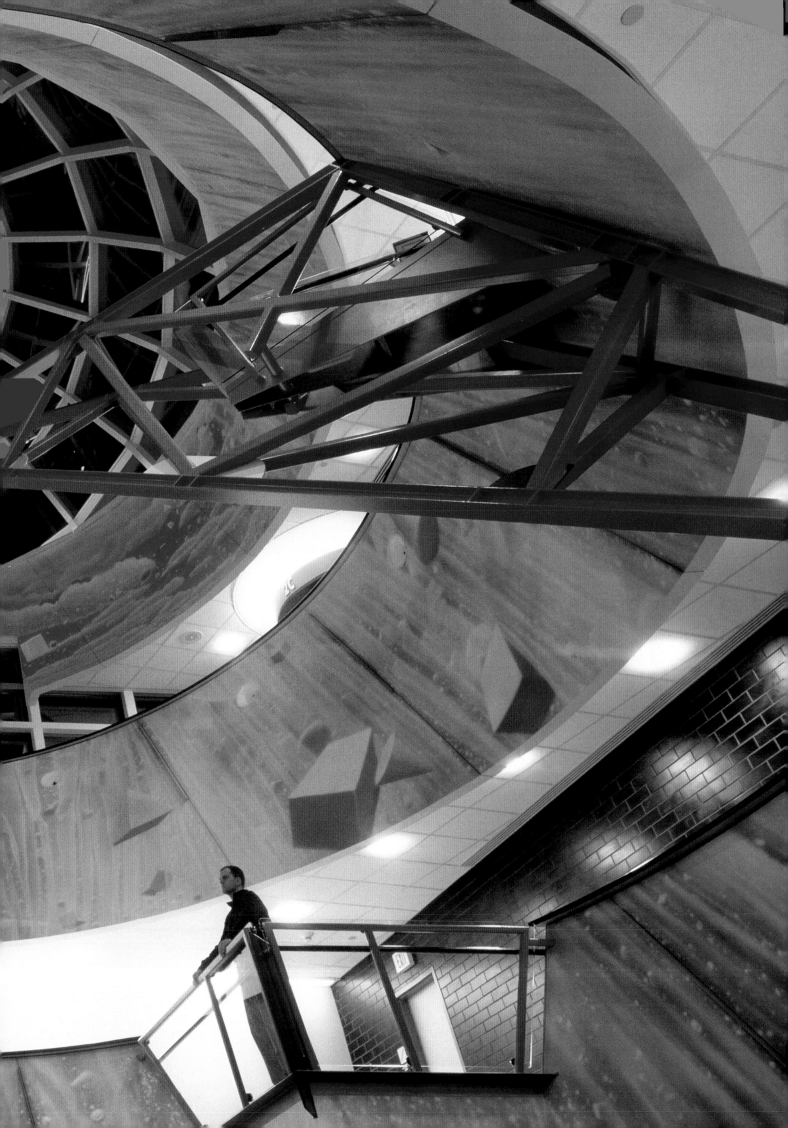

Connecticut Children's Hospital
Hartford, Connecticut, USA
HKS Inc.
Previous pages:
   Lobby/rotunda
Photo credit: Robert Benson Photography

Doernbecher Childrenís Hospital,
Oregon Health Sciences University
Portland, Oregon, USA
Zimmer Gunsul Frasca Partnership
in association with Anshen + Allen

1   Main Lobby
2   Three courtyards bring light into center of building
3   Orientation is clear with graphic signage and outdoor views
4   Meditation room provides a place of respite
5   Central nursing station serves a typical in-patient
     'neighbourhood'
6   Outpatient services are centralized on 7th level
7   Courtyards provide dedicated outdoor access areas for
     patients, families, visitors and staff
Photo credit: Eckert & Eckert Photographic (1,3–7);
Timothy Hursley (2)

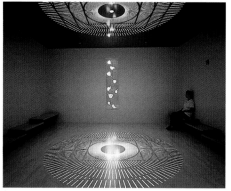

1

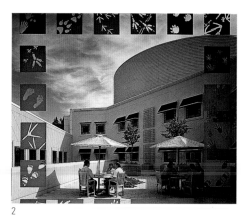

2

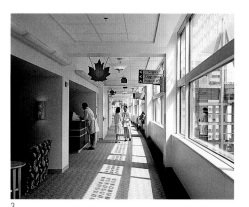

3

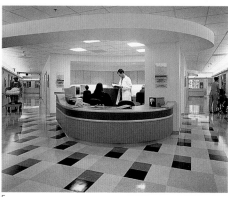

4

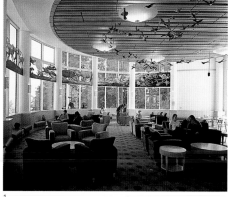

5

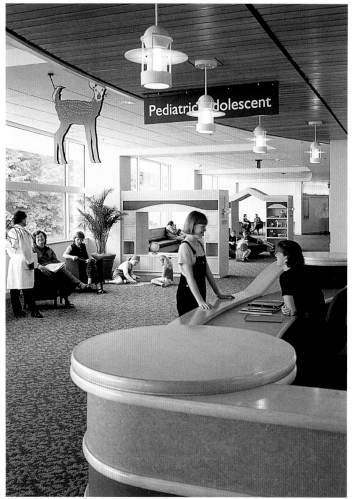

6

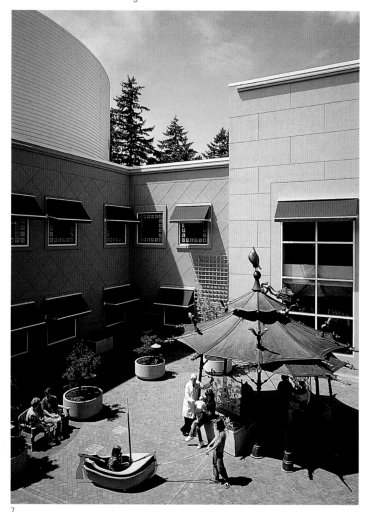

7

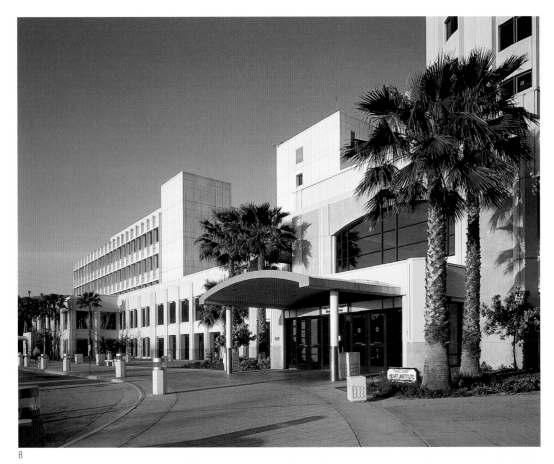

Loma Linda University Medical Center
Loma Linda, California, USA
NBBJ
8   Lobby and entrance to Cancer Research
      Institute
9   Courtyard area
Photo credit: Assassi Productions

8

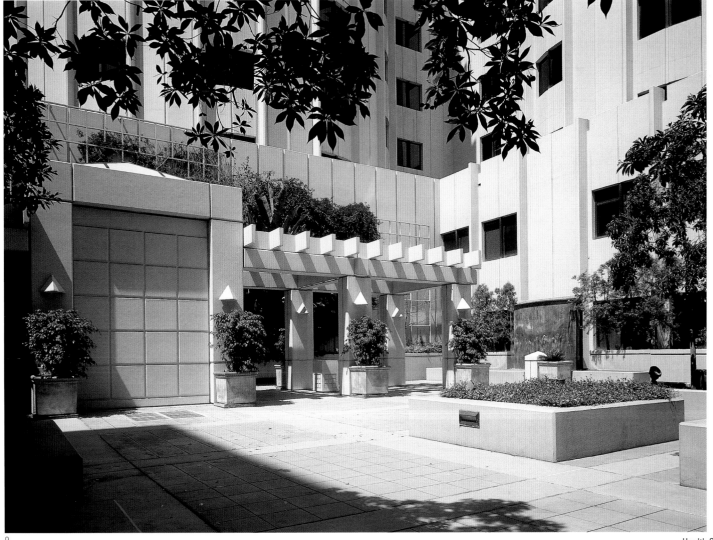

9

Vaasa Central Hospital
Vaasa, Finland
Paatela & Paatela Architects
1&2　Entrance of Emergency Department
　　　and Intensive Care Unit
Photo credit: Risto Laine

All Saints Episcopal Hospital
Fort Worth, Texas, USA
HKS Inc.
3　LDRP Patient room
Photo credit: Wes Thompson

Lutheran General Hospital
Park Ridge, Illinois, USA
Loebl Schlossman & Hackl
4　Simulator room
Opposite page:
　　Linear accelerator room
Photo credit: Bruce VanInwegen

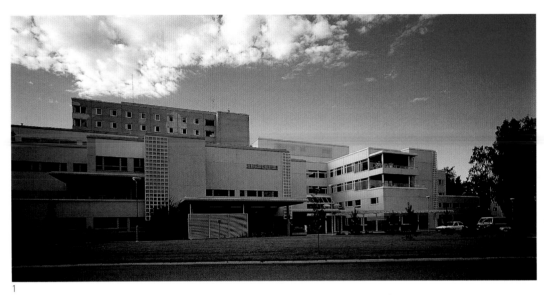

1

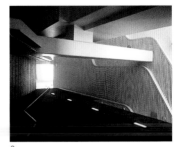

2

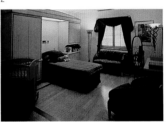

3

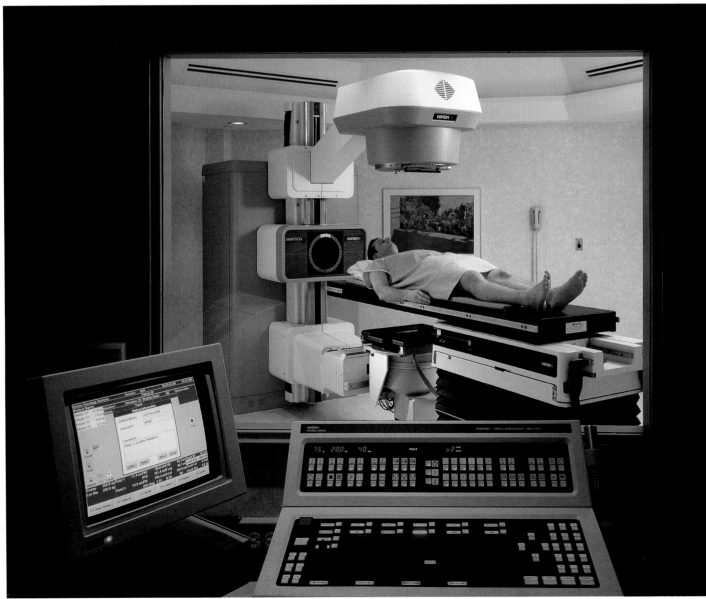

4

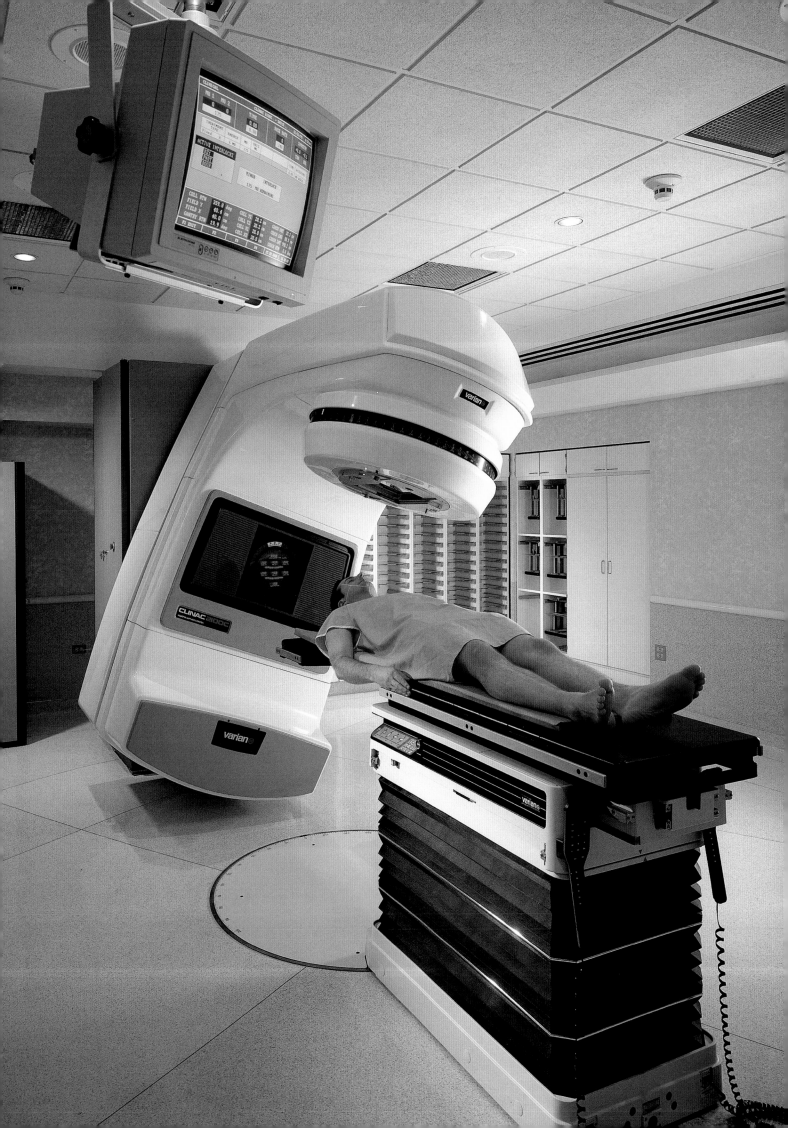

Rice Children's Center
Illinois, USA
Skidmore, Owings & Merrill LLP

1   Southern perspective from Bridge Avenue
2   South elevation of school wing
3   Interior view of school gymnasium
Photo credit: Hedrich-Blessing

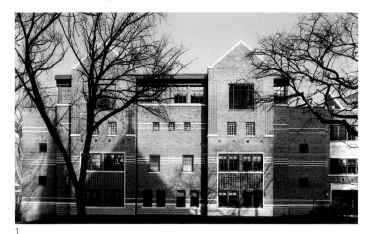

1

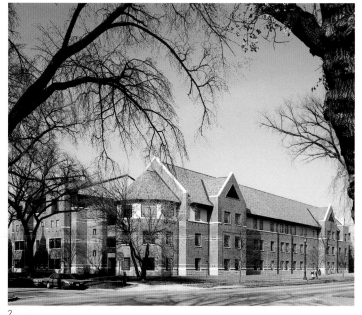

2

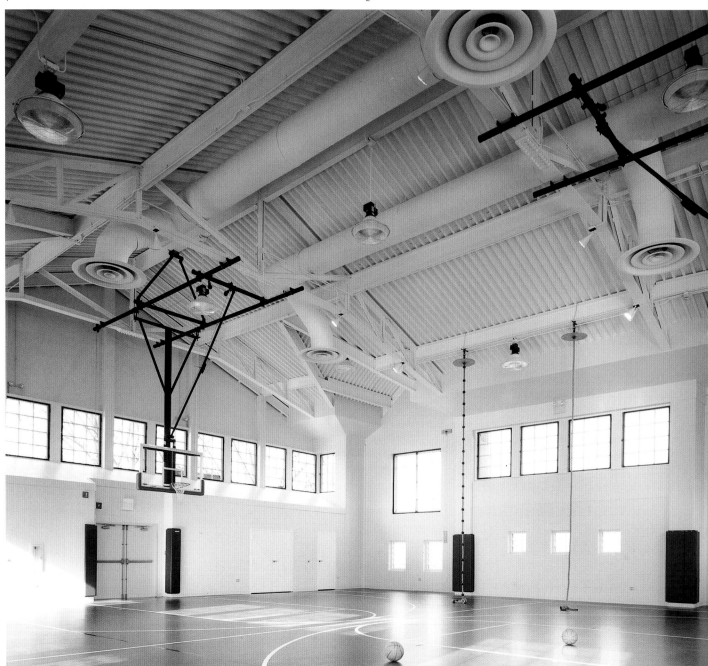

3

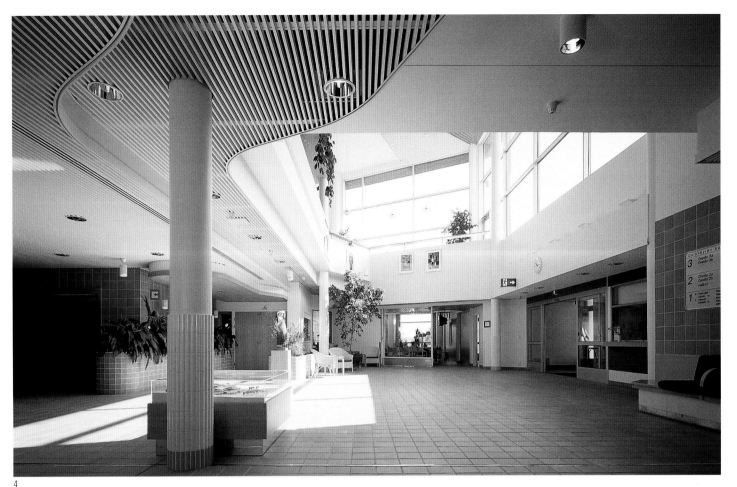

4

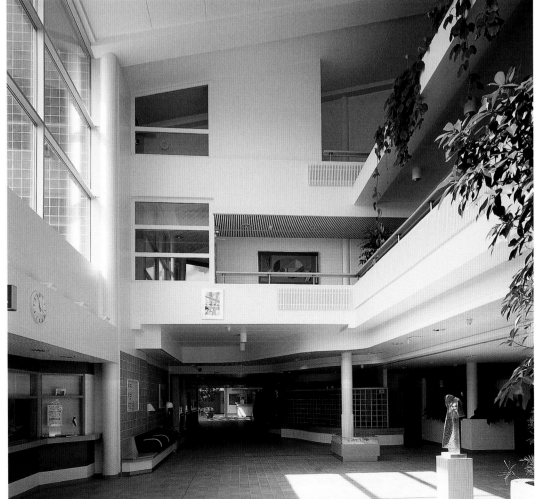

5

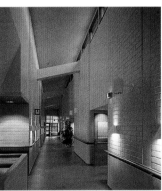

6

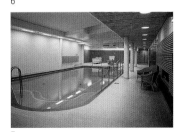

7

Oulunkylä Rehabilitation Hospital
Helsinki, Finland
Paatela & Paatela Architects

4&5   Entrance hall
  6   Corridor with roof lighting
  7   Swimming pool for rehabilitation
Photo credits: Gero Mylius (4); Timo Kauppila (5–7)

Barry Medical Park
Kansas City, Missouri, USA
WRS Architects Inc.

Following pages:
      State-of-the-art therapy gymnasium
      within Outpatient Rehabilitation Suite
Photo credit: Mike Sinclair Photography

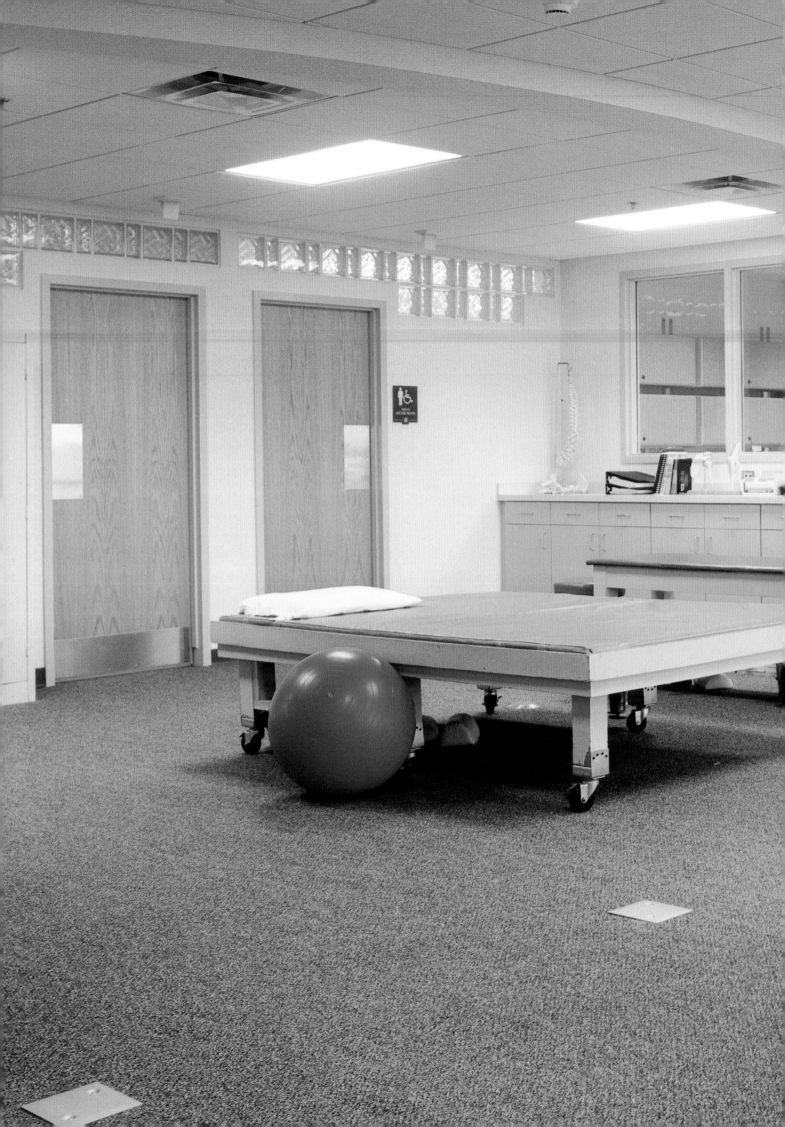

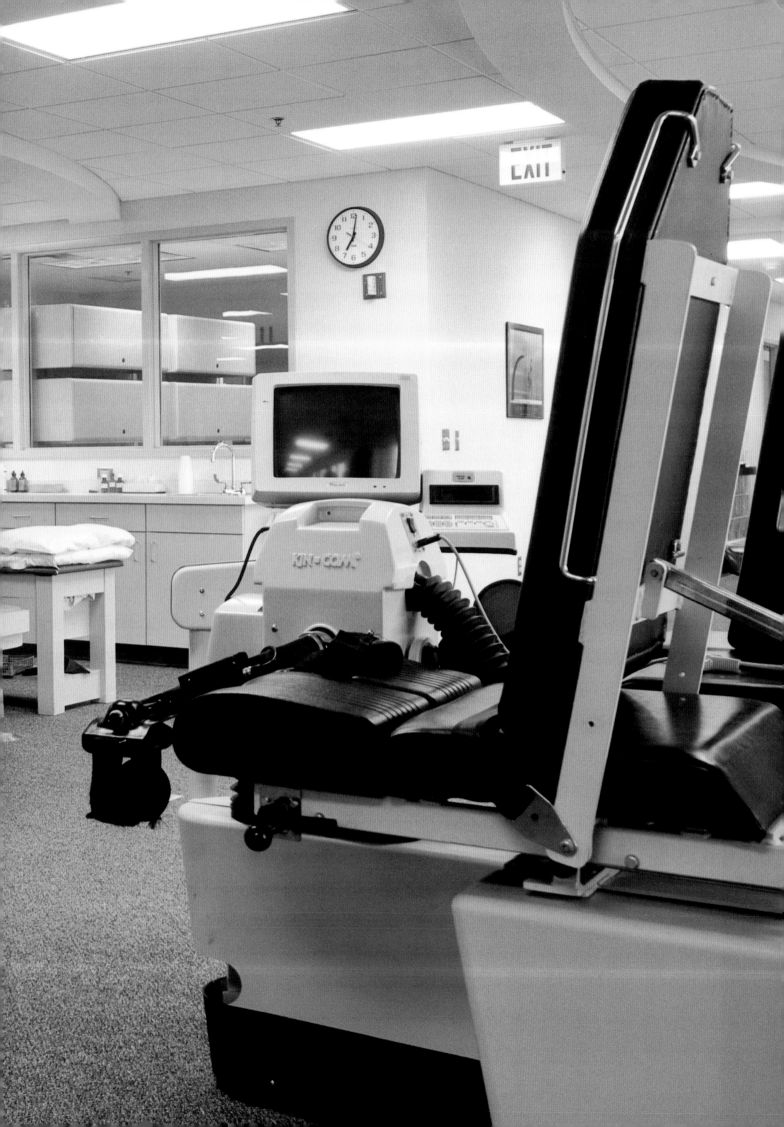

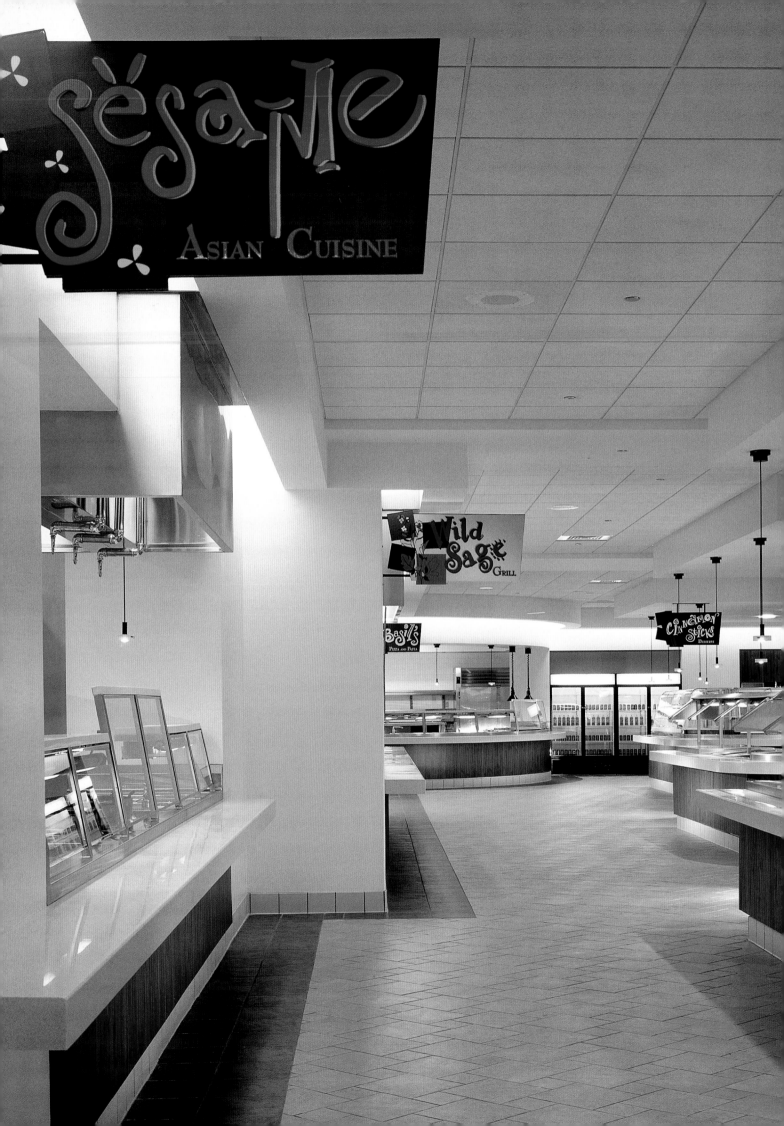

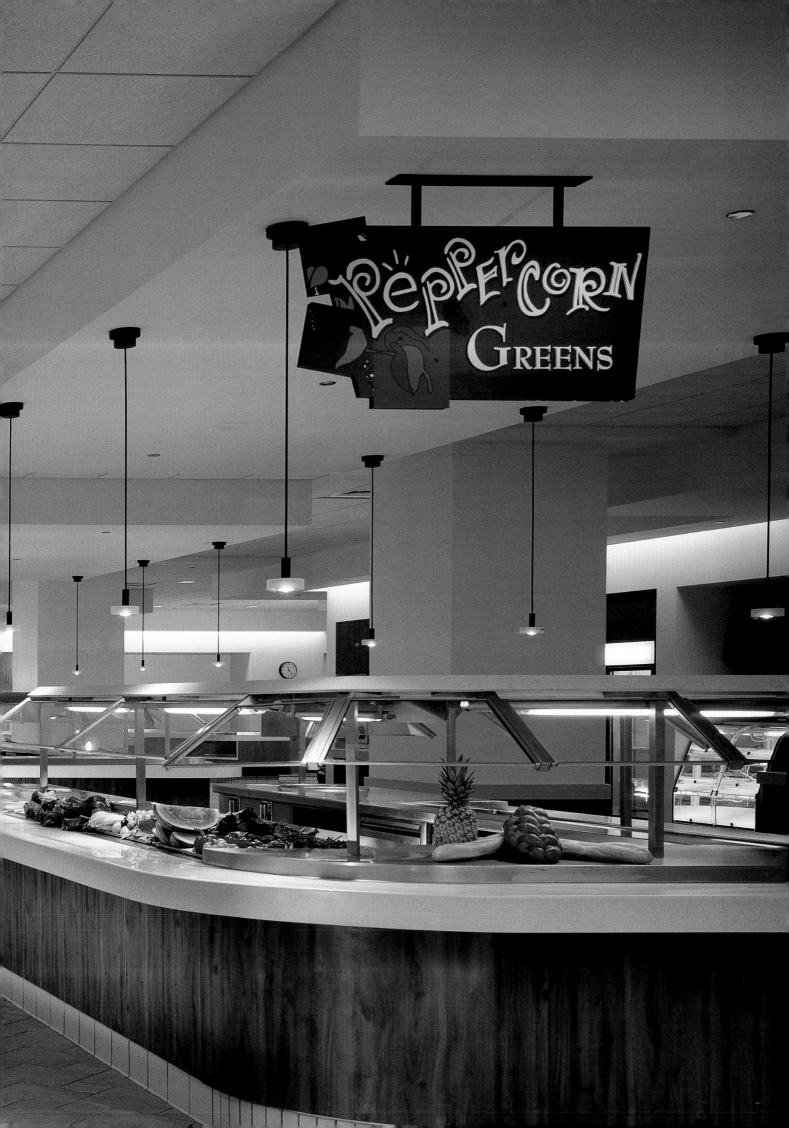

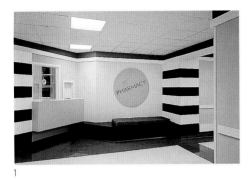

1

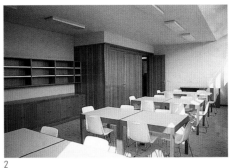

2

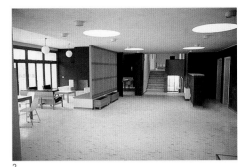

3

**Northwestern Memorial Hospital
Chicago, Illinois, USA**
Hellmuth, Obata + Kassabaum, Inc. in
association with Ellerbe Becket and VOA
Previous pages:
       Visitors eat at hotel-like cafeteria
Photo credit: Craig Dugan/Hedrich-Blessing

**Northeast Georgia Health Services–Short
Stay Surgery
Gainsville, Georgia, USA**
Quantrell Mullins & Associates Inc.
    1   Pharmacy
Photo credit: Brian Robbins

**Centro Diagnostico Neuro Psichiatrico
Imola, Bologna, Italy**
Enzo Zacchiroli Architetto
    2&3   Leisure space for creative activities
Photo credit: courtesy of Enzo Zacchiroli Architetto

**Utah Valley Regional Medical Center's
Women's and Children's Addition
Provo, Utah, USA**
HKS Inc. in association with Design West
    4   Public space
Photo credit: Ed LaCasse

**HealthPark Medical Center
Fort Myers, Florida, USA**
HKS Inc.
    5   Operating room
Photo credit: Rick Grumbaum

**University Center for Community Health
San Antonio, Texas, USA**
Marmon Mok
    6   View along renal dialysis building toward
         cafeteria and main building
    7   View of entry to an interior courtyard
    8   Stair tower as a symbolic marker for the
         presence of state-of-the–art medical care
Photo credit: C. Blackmon

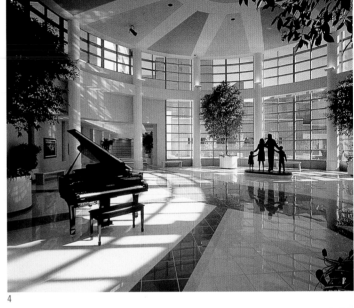

4

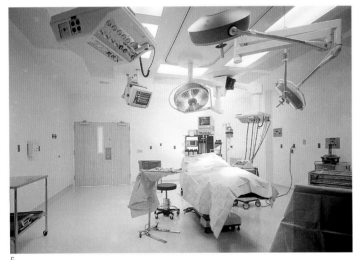

5

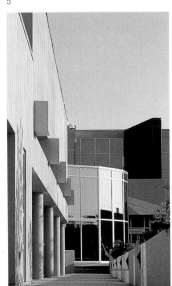

6

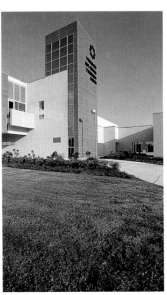

7

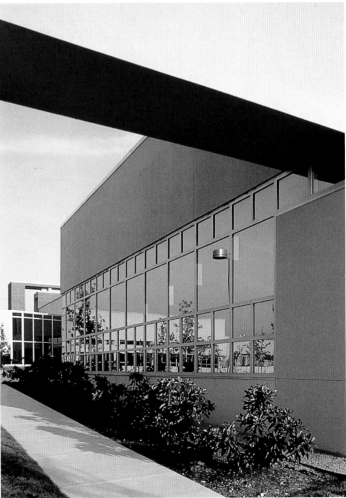

8

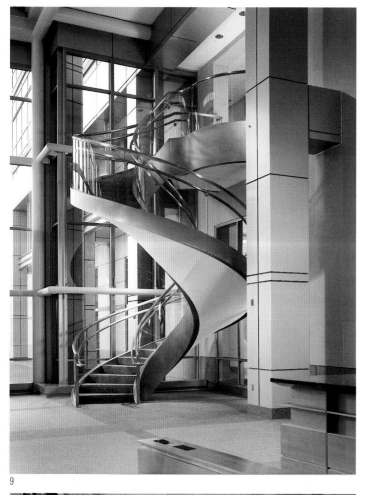

9

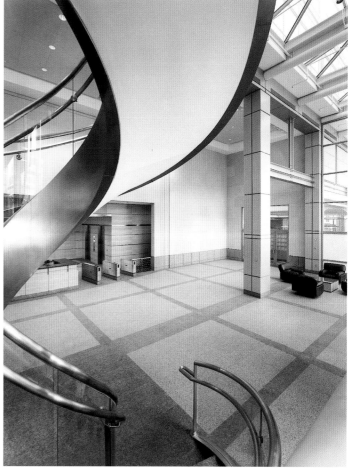

10

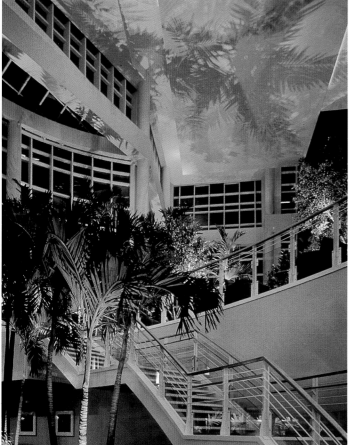

11

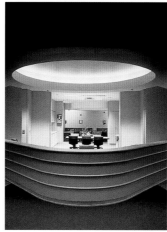

12

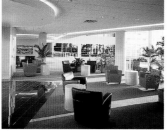

13

Children's Hospital of Philadelphia, Abramson Pediatric Research Center
Philadelphia, Pennsylvania, USA
Ellenzweig Associates, Inc.

9   Lobby stair
10   View of curved stairwell with waiting
        area in background
Photo credit: Tom Crane

Health Central
Ocoee, Florida, USA
HKS Inc.

11   Night view of atrium
12   Patient care unit nurses' station/
        reception
13   Colourful, second-floor patient care
        unit, waiting area
Photo credit: Rick Grumbaum & Michael Lowry

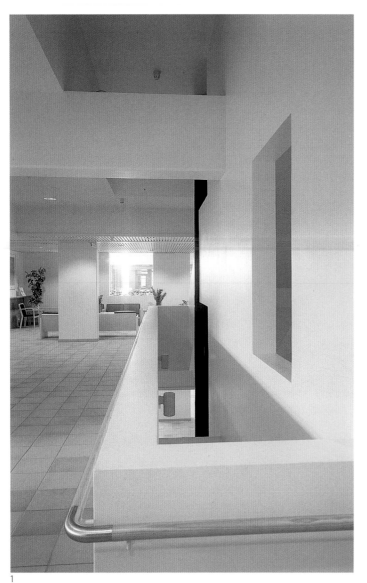

1

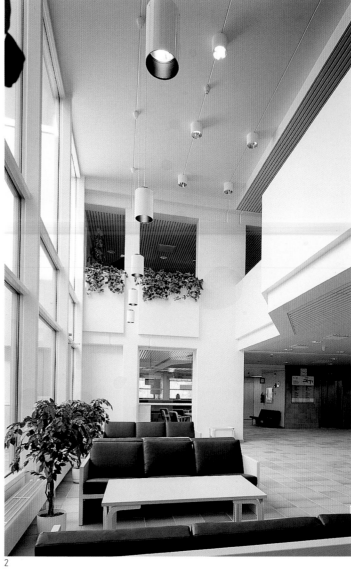

2

**Helsinki University Central Hospital for
Skin and Allergic Diseases
Helskini, Finland**
Paatela & Paatela Architects
1   Detail of staircase with waiting area in
    background
2   Two-storey main lobby
3   Inner courtyard
Photo credits: Timo Kauppila

**Loma Linda University Medical Center
Loma Linda, California, USA**
NBBJ
4   Play area at Children's Hospital
5   Waiting area for Proton Beam Therapy
    facility
6   Lobby and entrance to Cancer Research
    Institute
Photo credits: courtesy of NBBJ (4);
David Wakely (5); Assassi Productions (6)

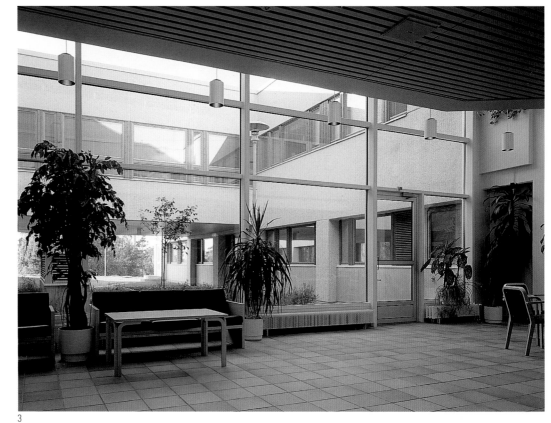

3

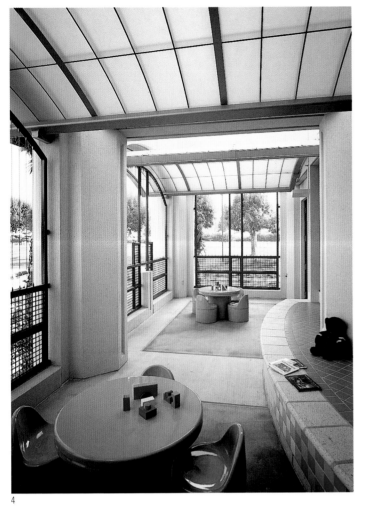

4

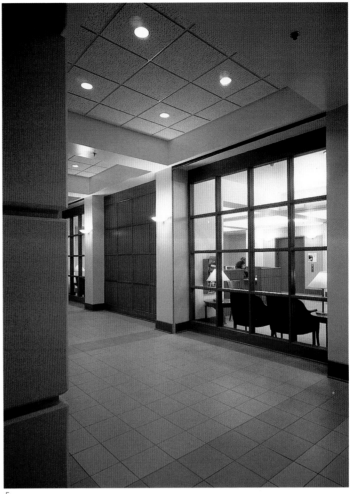

5

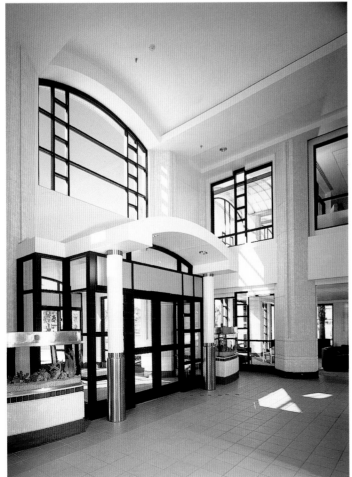

6

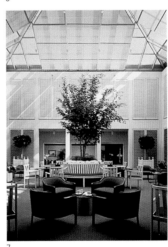

7

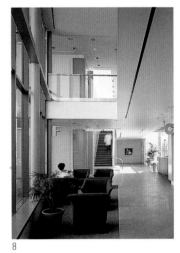

8

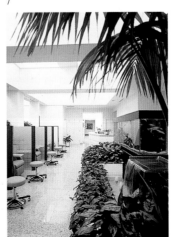

9

Milstein Pavilion, Presbyterian Hospital
Manhattan, New York, USA
Skidmore, Owings & Merrill LLP
7   Private patient unit atrium
Photo credit: courtesy of Skidmore, Owings &
Merrill LLP

Kaiser Vallejo Office Building
Vallejo, California, USA
Skidmore, Owings & Merrill LLP
8   Main circulation spine
Photo credit: courtesy of Skidmore, Owings &
Merrill LLP

Schumpert Cancer Center
Shreveport, Louisiana, USA
HKS Inc.
9   Infusion therapy area
Photo credit: Rick Grumbaum

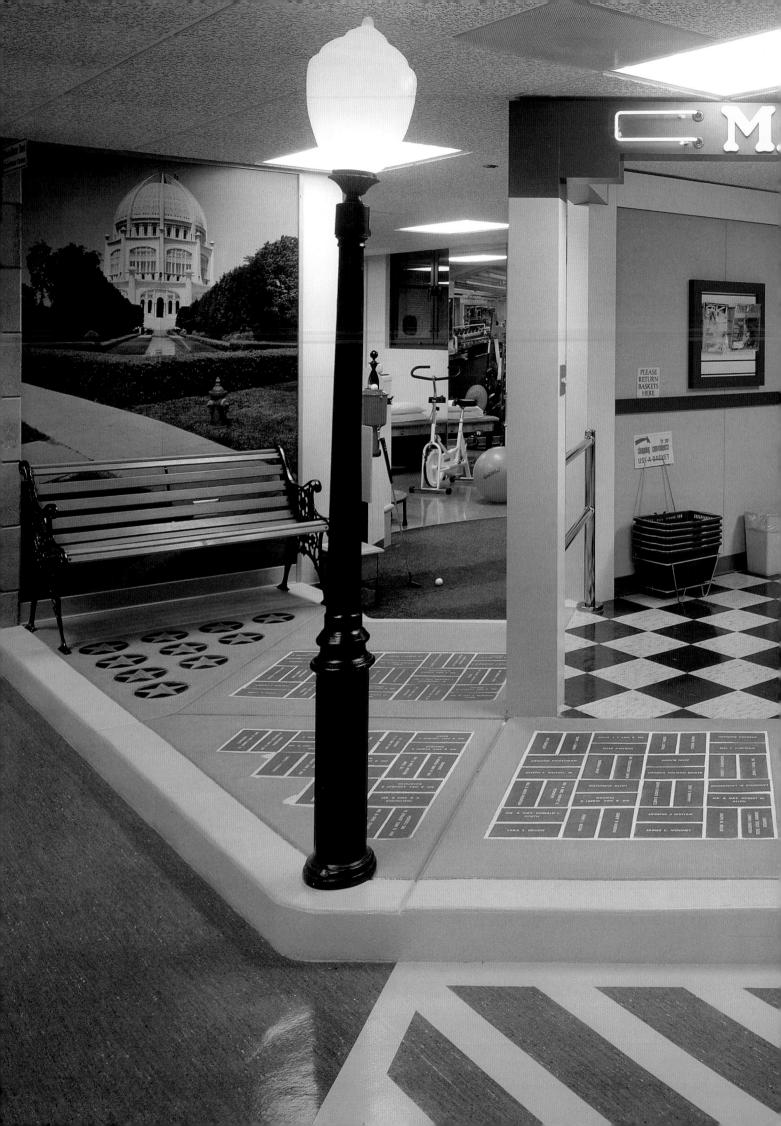

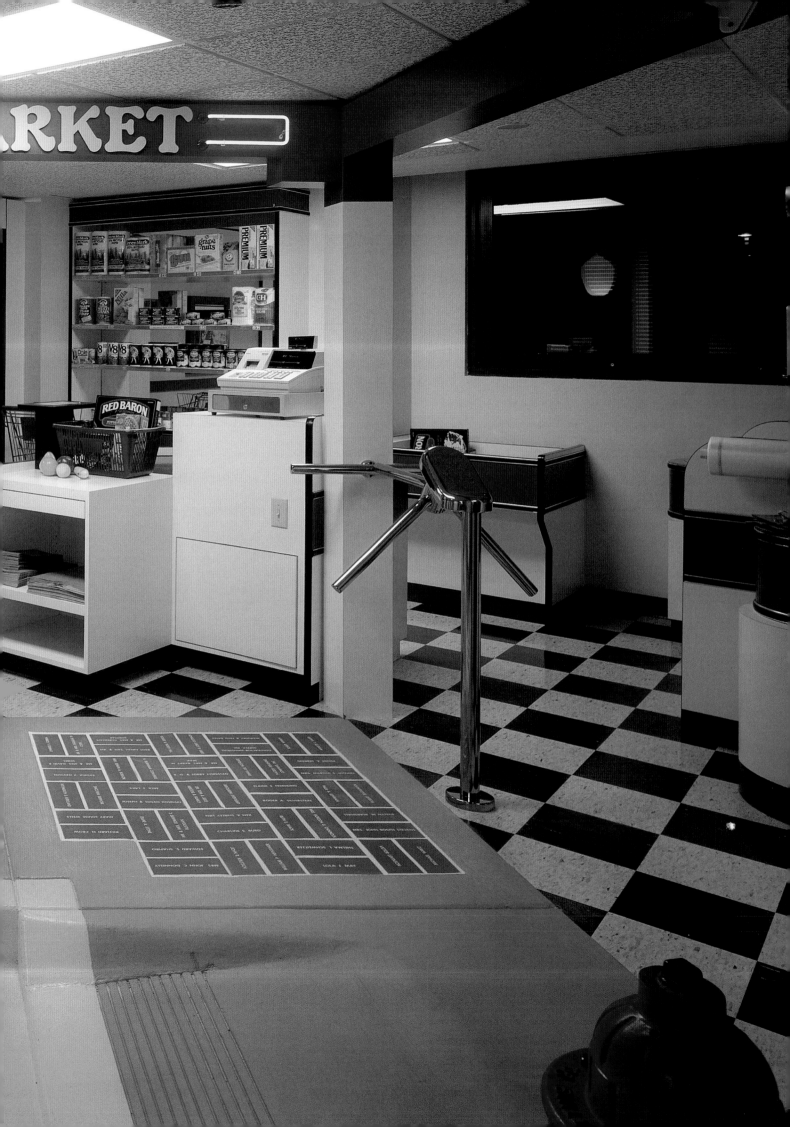

Evanston Hospital
Evanston, Illinois, USA
Loebl Schlossman & Hackl
Previous pages:
   'Easy Street' entrance—rehabilitation
   patient's therapy takes them through this
   neon-lit, fully stocked grocery store.
Photo credit: Judy A. Slagle

Beth Israel Hospital & Children's Hospital,
Medical Care Center
Lexington, Massachusetts, USA
Steffian Bradley Associates, Inc.
1   View from surgery waiting area to atrium
Photo credit: Wayne Soverns Jr.

Valley Children's Hospital
Madera, California, USA
HKS Inc.
2   Patient room
3   Paediatric Intensive Care Unit
Photo credit: Kelly Petersen

Evanston Hospital
Evanston, Illinois, USA
Loebl Schlossman & Hackl
4   Medical records—reception area
5   Medical records—work area
Photo credit: Bruce VanInwegen

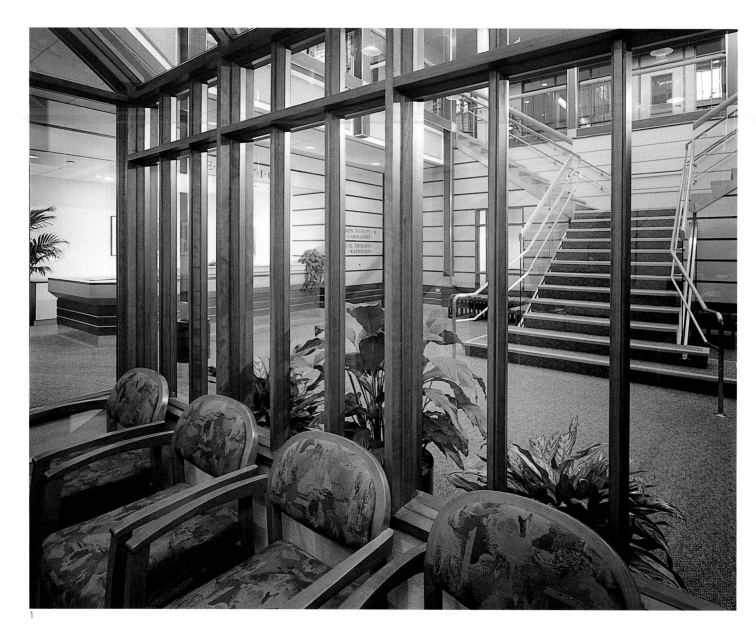

1

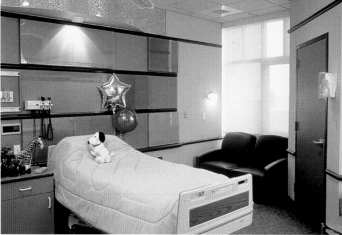

2

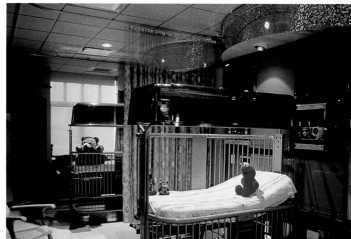

3

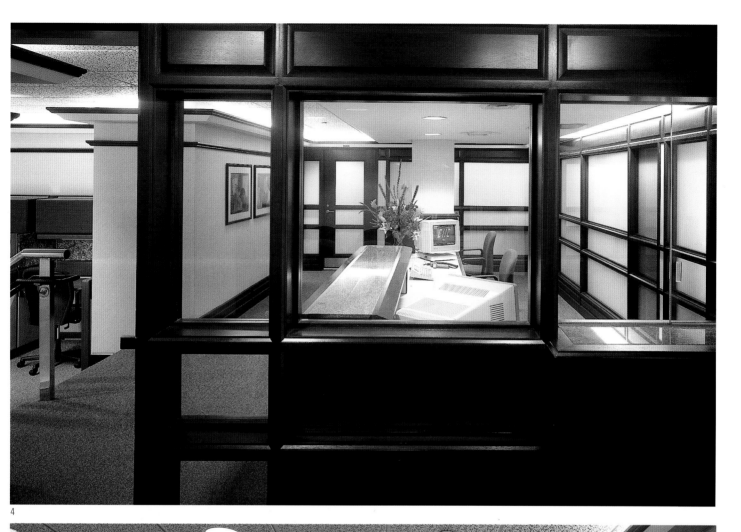

4

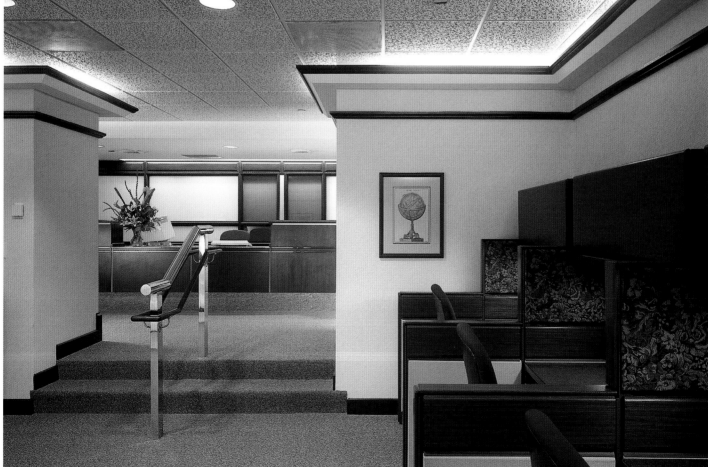

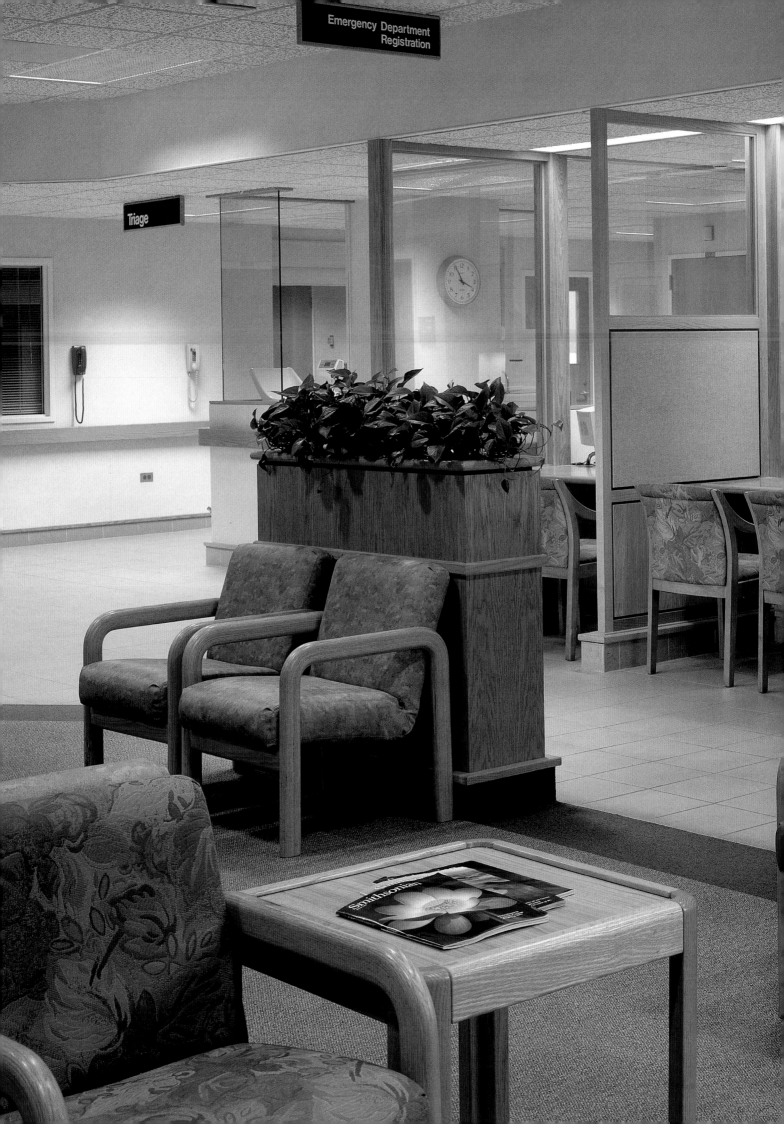

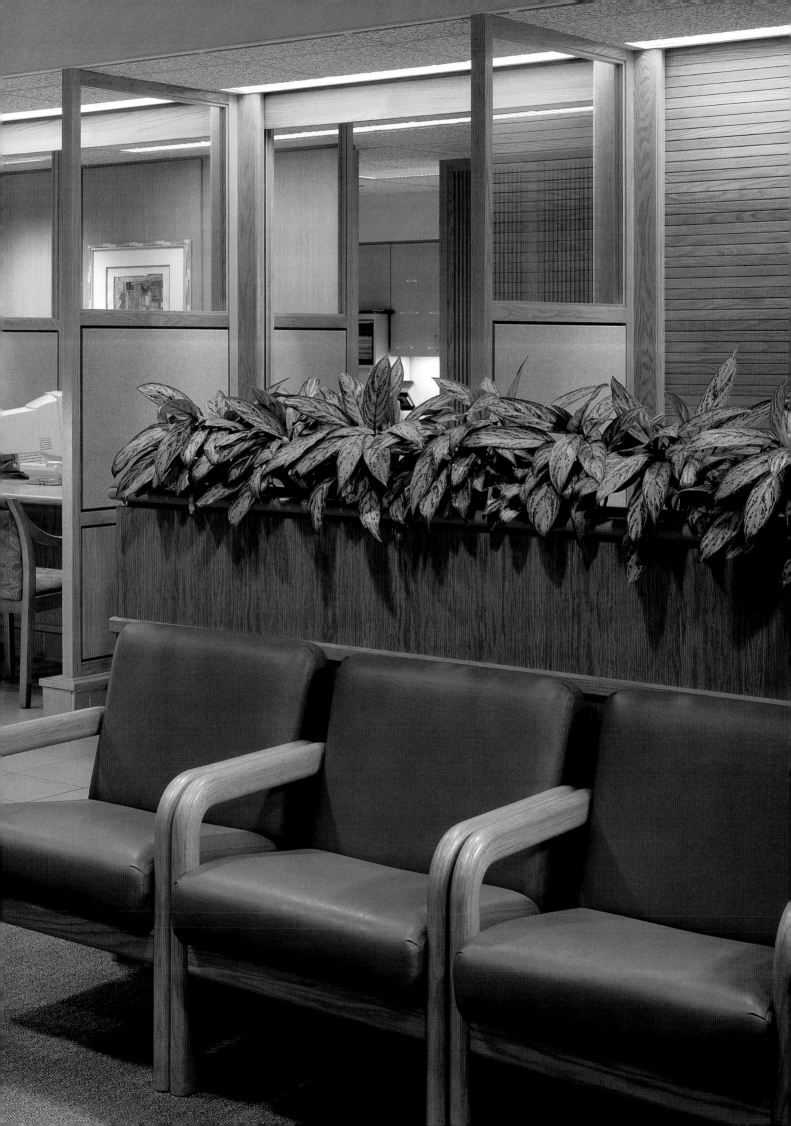

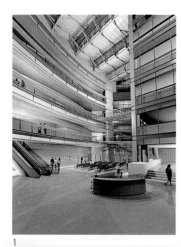

1

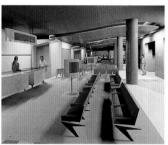

2

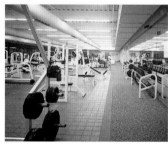

3

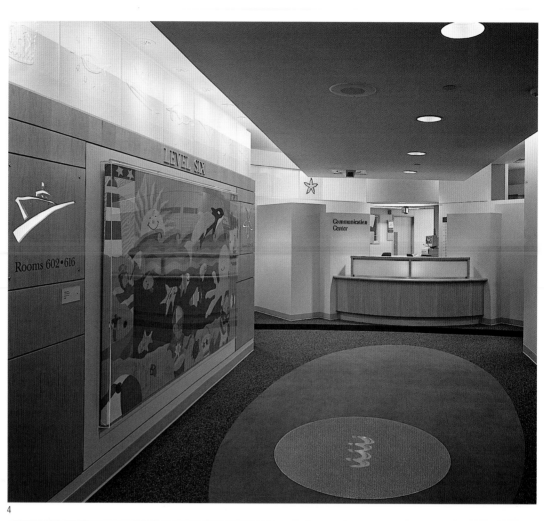

4

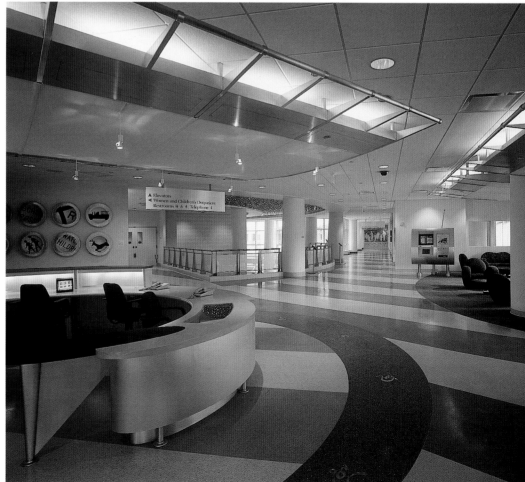

5

Evanston Hospital
Evanston, Illinois, USA
Loebl Schlossman & Hackl
Previous pages:
    Emergency Department's waiting area
Photo credit: Bruce VanInwegen

Kangbuk Samsung Medical Center
Seoul, Korea
NBBJ
1   Main lobby
2   Waiting area
Photo credit: courtesy of NBBJ

Rex Primary Care and Wellness Center
Cary, North Carolina, USA
HKS Inc.
3   Fitness room
Photo credit: Jim Sink

Rainbow Babies and Children's Hospital
Cleveland, Ohio, USA
NBBJ
4   Elevator lobby
5   Main reception and waiting area
6   Animated finishes indicate many
     different play areas
Photo credit: Timothy Hursley

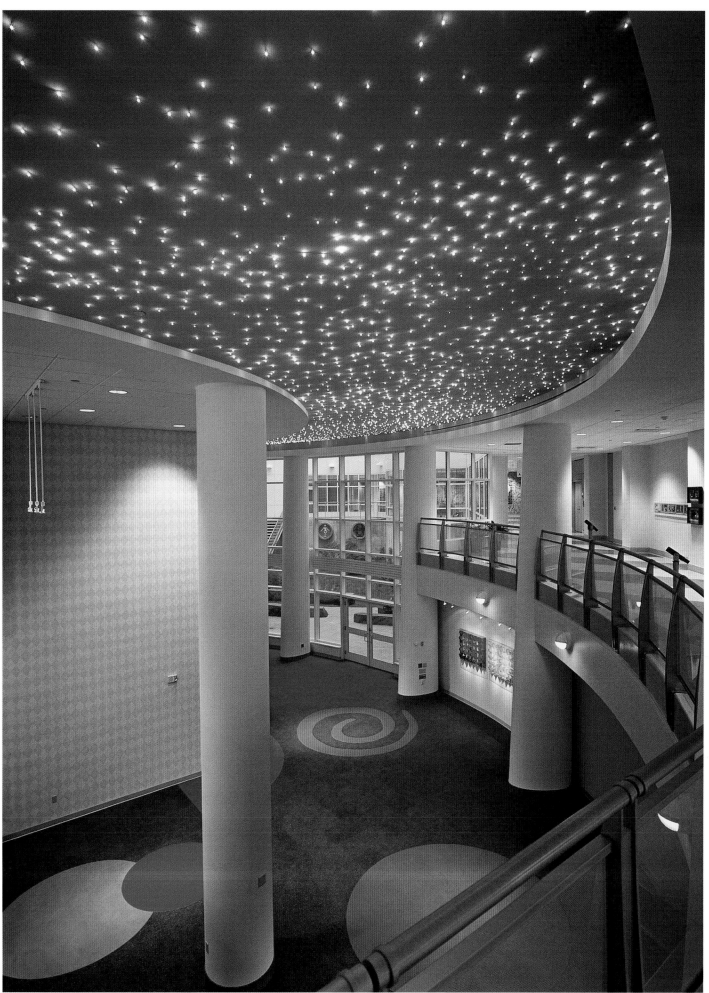

The New York Hospital
New York, USA
Hellmuth, Obata + Kassabaum, Inc.

1   Nursery
2   Paediatric playroom
3   Labour and delivery room
Photo credit: courtesy of Hellmuth, Obata + Kassabaum, Inc.

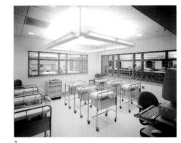

1

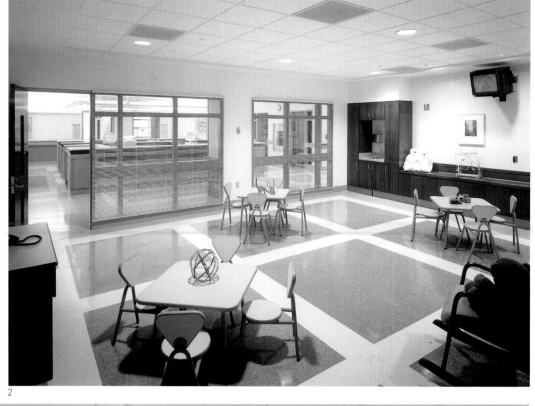

2

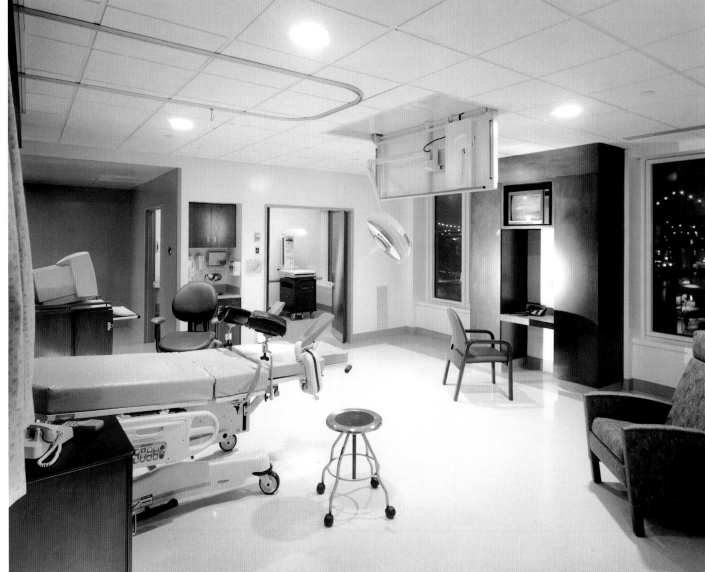

3

**University of Wisconsin Hospital &
Clinics–West Clinic
Madison, Wisconsin, USA**
Flad & Associates

4   Glass curtainwall allows daylight to fill
    waiting areas
5   Two-storey drum atrium marks single
    public entrance
6   Registration hub is the patient's first stop
7   Distinctive lighting and floor elements
    mark intersections and doorways
8   Exam rooms have windows with privacy
    control and high clerestory
Photo credit: Christopher Barrett

**St. Michael's Hospital
Stevens Point, Wisconsin, USA**
Flad & Associates

9   Chemotherapy treatment room focuses
    on privacy and peace
Photo credit: Christopher Barrett

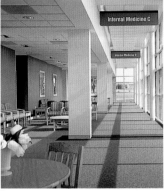

4

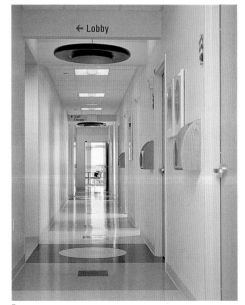

5

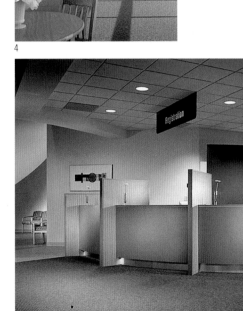

6

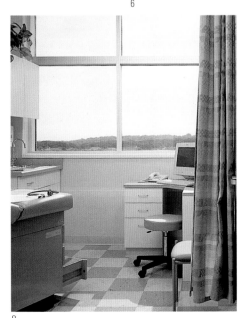

7

8

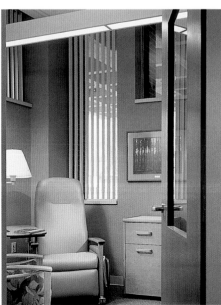

9

**Ontario Cancer Institute,
Princess Margaret Hospital
Toronto, Canada**
Hellmuth, Obata + Kassabaum, Inc.
1   Juice bar
2   Library
Photo credit: courtesy of Hellmuth, Obata
+ Kassabaum, Inc.

**Grossman Cancer Center, Cancer Therapy
& Research Center
San Antonio, Texas, USA**
Marmon Mok
3   Building lobby at radiotherapy floor
4   View of radiation therapy nurses' station
5   View from building lobby toward radiation
    therapy waiting area
6   View of main entry wall, fondly named
    'boomerang wall'
7   View of main entry and lobbies at dusk
8   View up at building's spatially dramatic
    four-storey lobby
Photo credits: Aker/Zvonkovic (3,4,7,8); courtesy of
Marmon Mok (5&6)

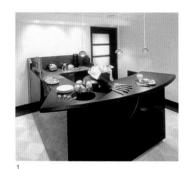

1

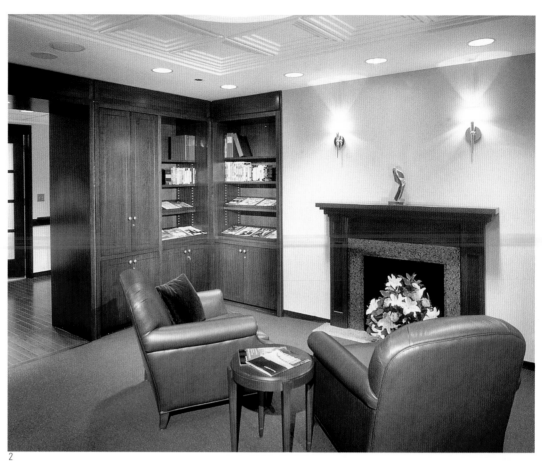

2

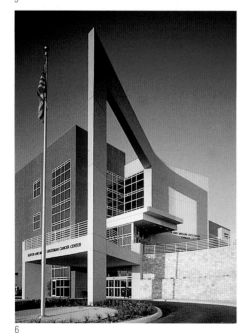

3

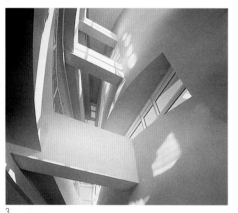

4

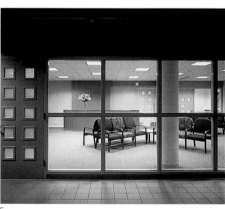

5

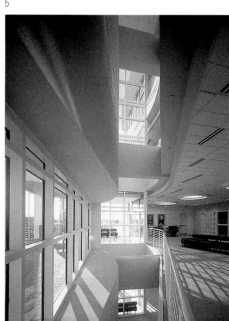

6

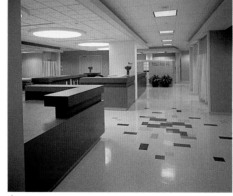

7

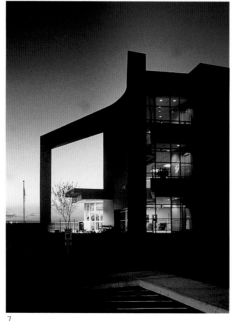

8

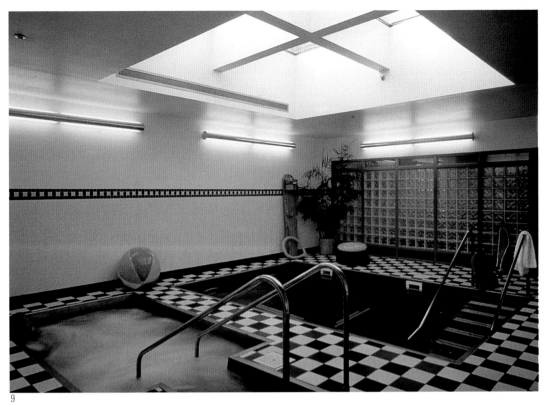

All Saints Episcopal Hospital
Fort Worth, Texas, USA
HKS Inc.

9   Rehabilitation and Wellness Center
Photo credit: Wes Thompson

Menninger Foundation
Topeka, Kansas, USA
Skidmore, Owings & Merrill LLP

10   Psychiatric unit building
Photo credit: courtesy of Skidmore, Owings &
Merrill LLP

Community Health Services
Connecticut, USA
Du Bose Associates, Inc., Architects

11   Warm colours, ample daylight and wood
      humanize main waiting area
Photo credit: Robert Benson Photography

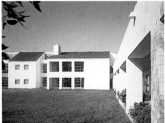

9

10

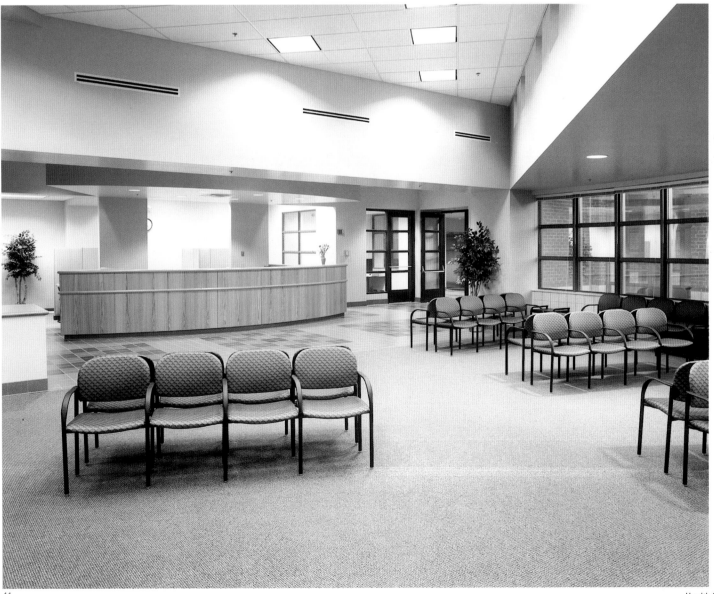

11

**Edward Health and Fitness Centre
at Seven Bridges
Woodridge, Illinois, USA**
Phillips Swager Associates
1   Track
2   Overview of workout area
4   Lap and therapy pool
5   Aerobics room
Photo credit: Barry Rustin Photography

**Grossman Cancer Center,
Cancer Therapy & Research Center
San Antonio, Texas, USA**
Marmon Mok
3   View of building's northwest elevation
     including entry plaza
Photo credit: courtesy of Marmon Mok

**MD Anderson Cancer Center
Houston, Texas, USA**
LAN/HKS Inc. Joint Venture
6   MRI
7   Linear accelerator
Photo credit: Wes Thompson (6); Michael Lowry (7)

**Northwestern Memorial Hospital
Chicago, Illinois, USA**
Hellmuth, Obata + Kassabaum, Inc. in
association with Ellerbe Becket and VOA
Opposite:
     Public spaces are comfortable and warm
Photo credit: Justin Machonochie/Hedrich-
Blessing

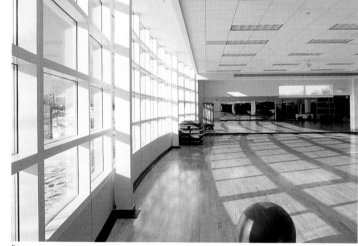

1

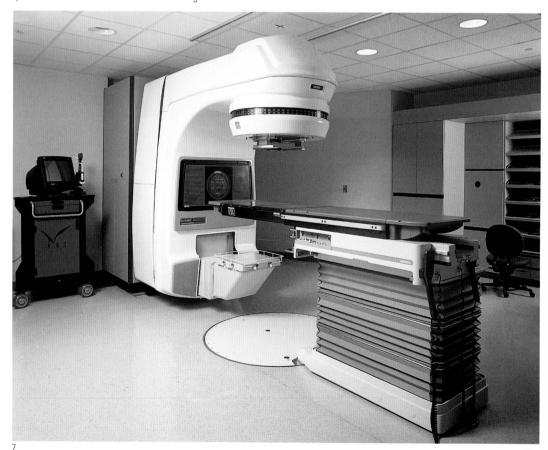

2

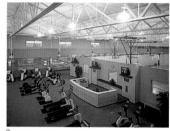

3

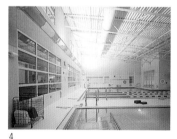

4

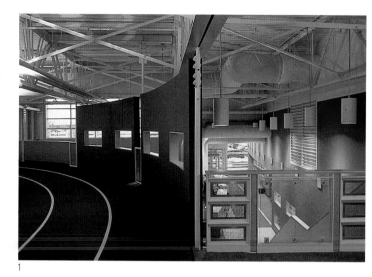

5

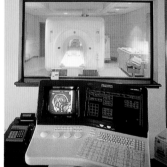

6

7

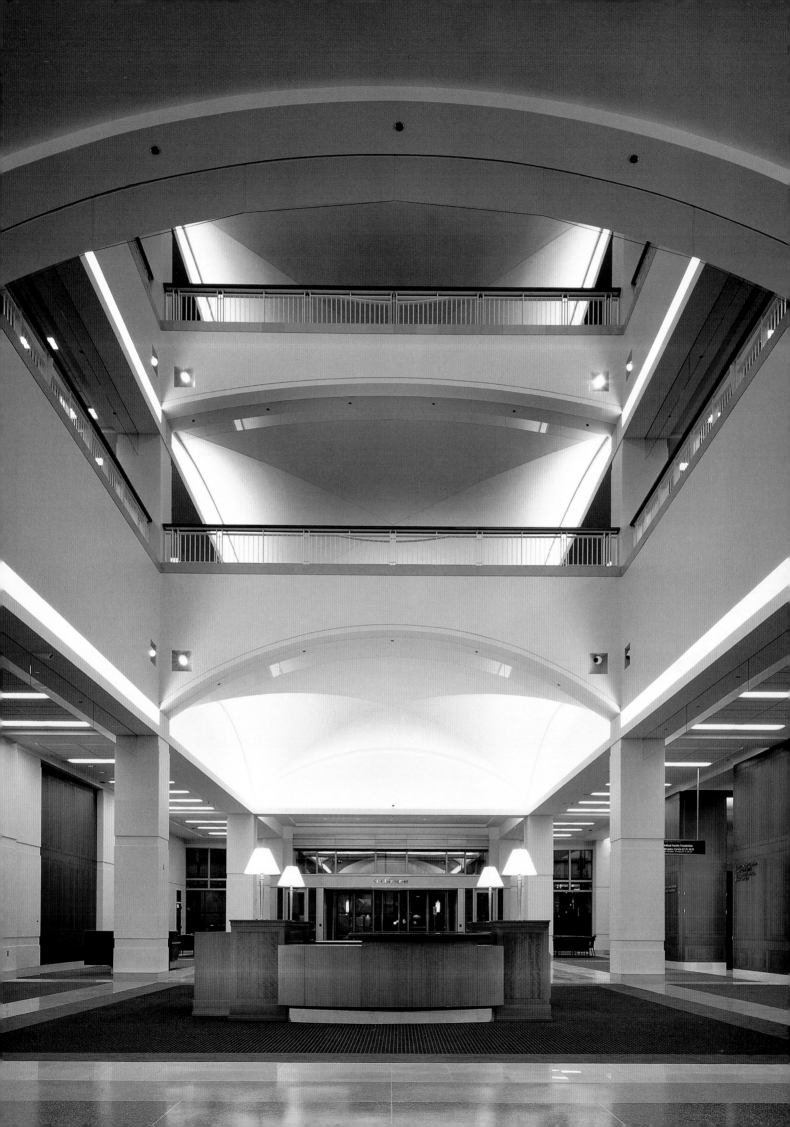

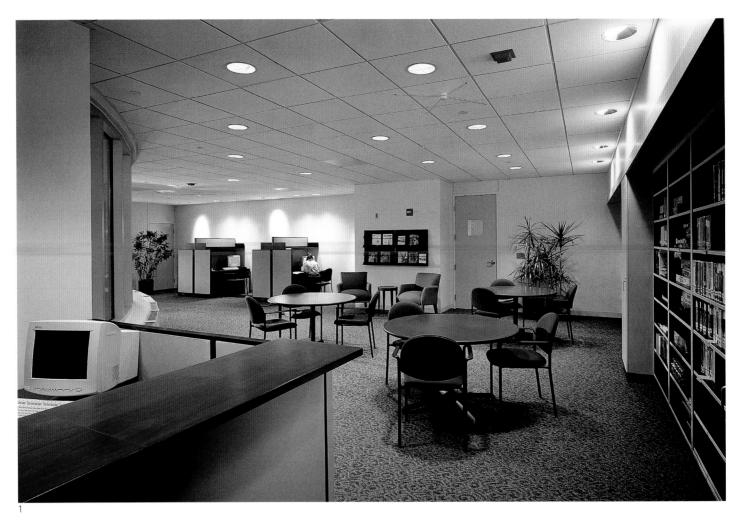

1

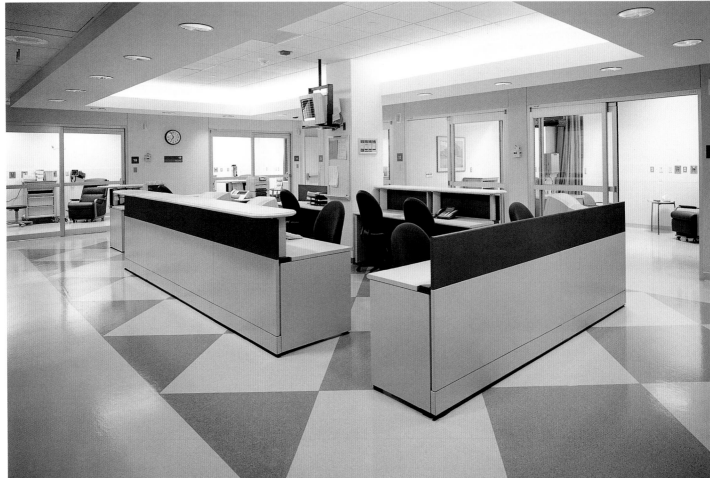

2

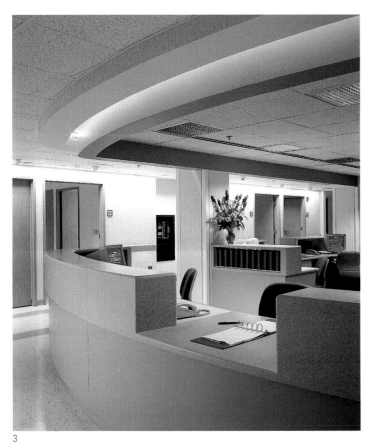

**University of Nebraska,
Lied Transplant Center
Omaha, Nebraska, USA**
Hellmuth, Obata + Kassabaum, Inc. in
association with Leo A Daly
1   Research and Information Center
2   Nurses' station in Treatment Center
Photo credit: Paul Brokering

**Hinsdale Hospital
Hinsdale, Illinois, USA**
Loebl Schlossman & Hackl
3&5   Cardiac Care Unit–nurses' station
Photo credit: Bruce VanInwegen

**Vaasa Central Hospital
Vaasa, Finland**
Paatela & Paatela Architects
4   Central lobby
Photo credit: courtesy of Paatela & Paatela
Architects

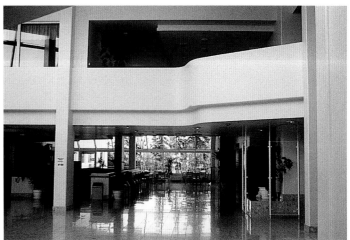

3

4

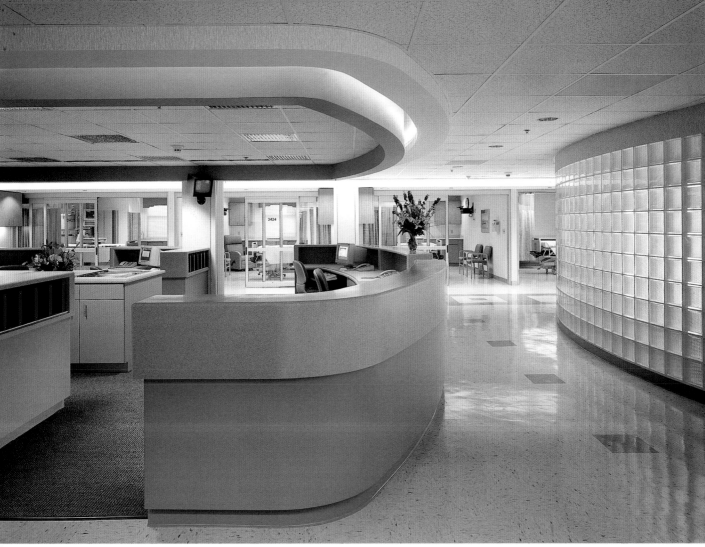

5

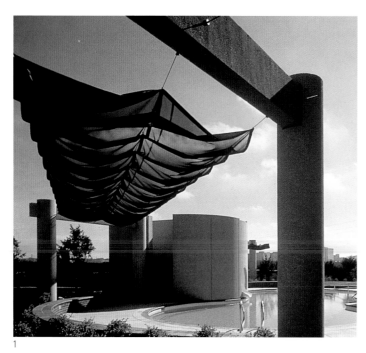

1

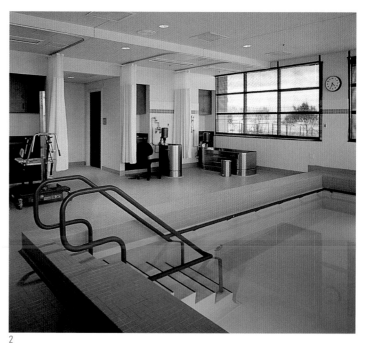

2

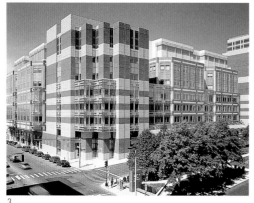

3

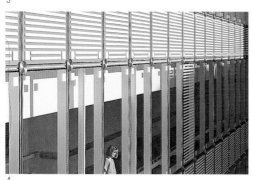

4

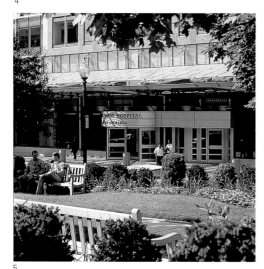

5

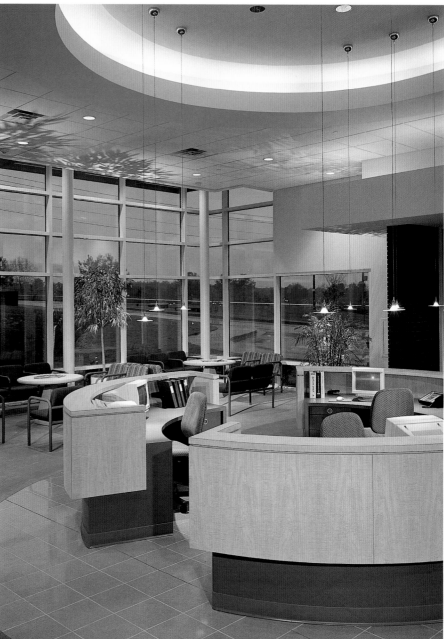

6

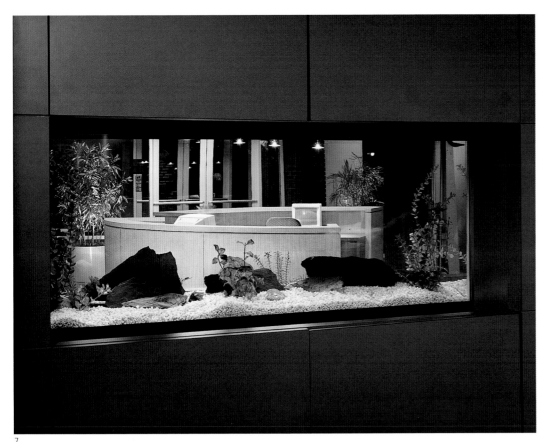

7

Warm Springs Rehabilitation Hospital
San Antonio, Texas, USA
HKS Inc.
1   Therapy pool
2   Hydrotherapy area
Photo credit: Rick Grumbaum

Beth Israel Deaconess Medical Center
Boston, Massachusetts, USA
Shepley Bulfinch Richardson and Abbott
3   Building overlooks new 'heart of the
     institution', a garden
4   Public concourse connecting bridge links
     campus buildings
5   Exterior view of glass canopy
Photo credit: Richard Mandelkorn

Prudential Health Care System HMO
Lithonia, Georgia, USA
Quantrell Mullins & Associates Inc.
6   Waiting area
7   View of reception through fish tank
8   Nurses' station and waiting area
Photo credit: Brian Robbins

Olympia Medical Center, Group Health
Cooperative of Puget Sound
Olympia, Washington, USA
Zimmer Gunsul Frasca Partnership
9   Main lobby maximizes natural light
10   Main entry stair looking south
Photo credit: Strode Eckert Photographic

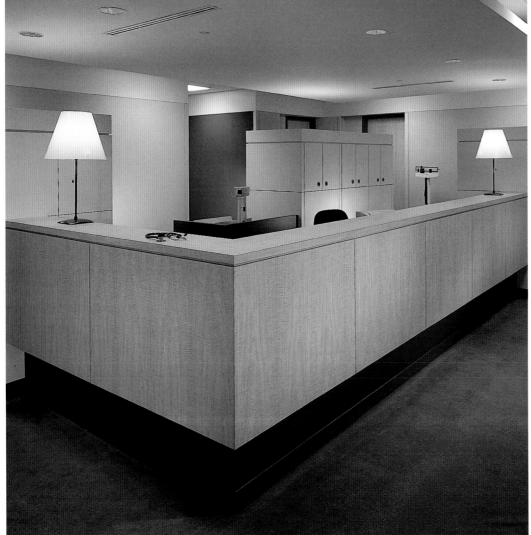

8

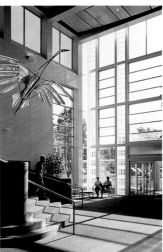

9

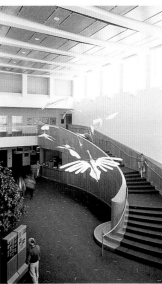

10

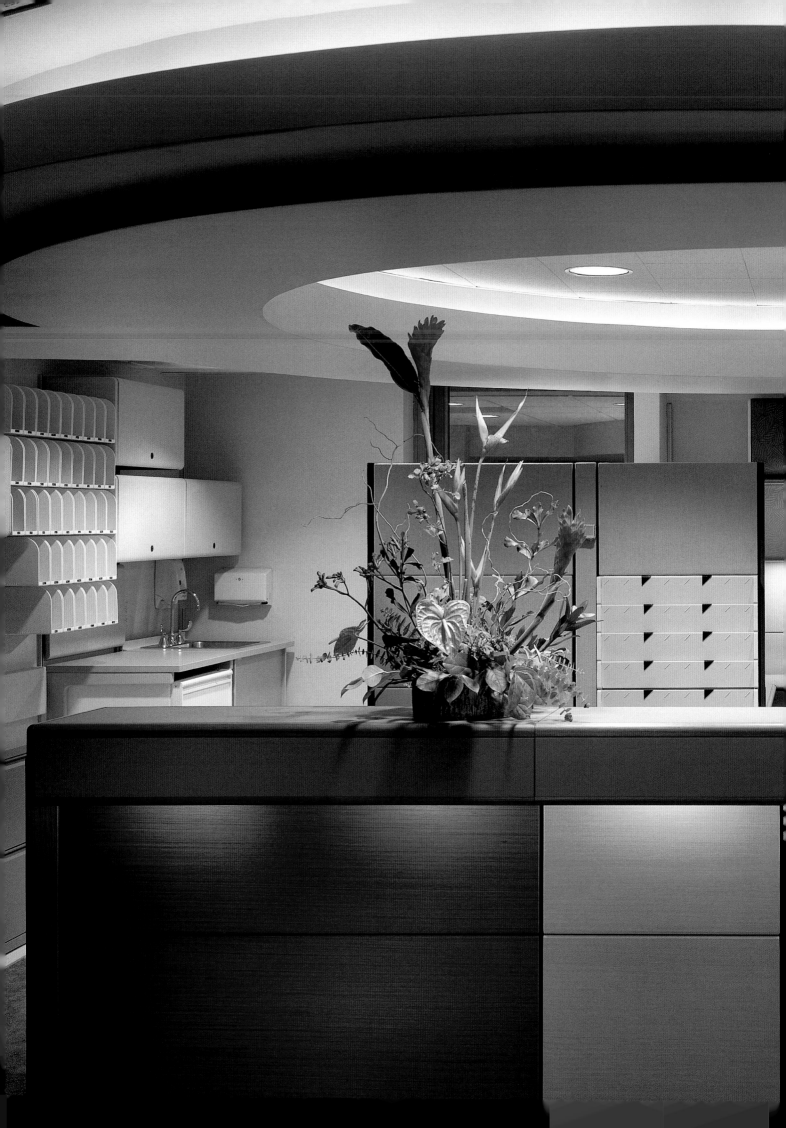

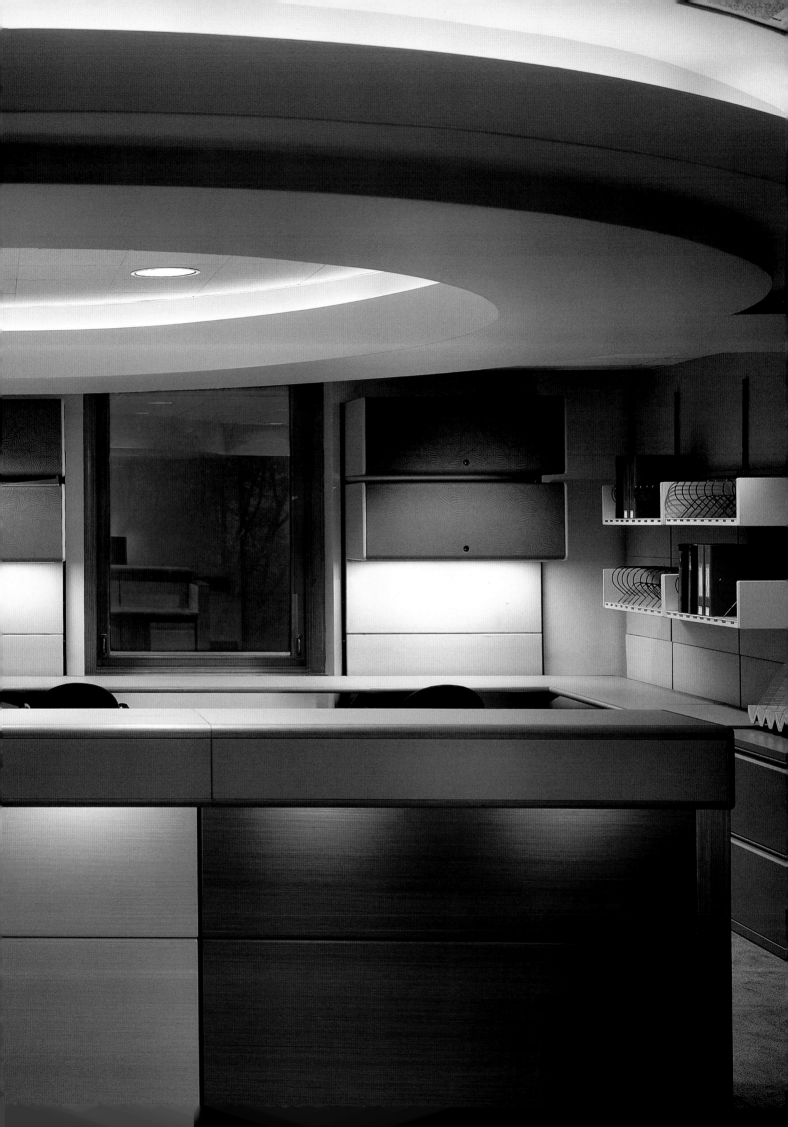

Resurrection Medical Center
Chicago, Illinois, USA
Loebl Schlossman & Hackl

Previous pages:
    Second floor nurses' station
1   Radiology Department's reception lobby and waiting area
2   Radiology Department's waiting area
3   Emergency Department's nurses' station with treatment room in background
Photo credit: Bruce VanInwegen

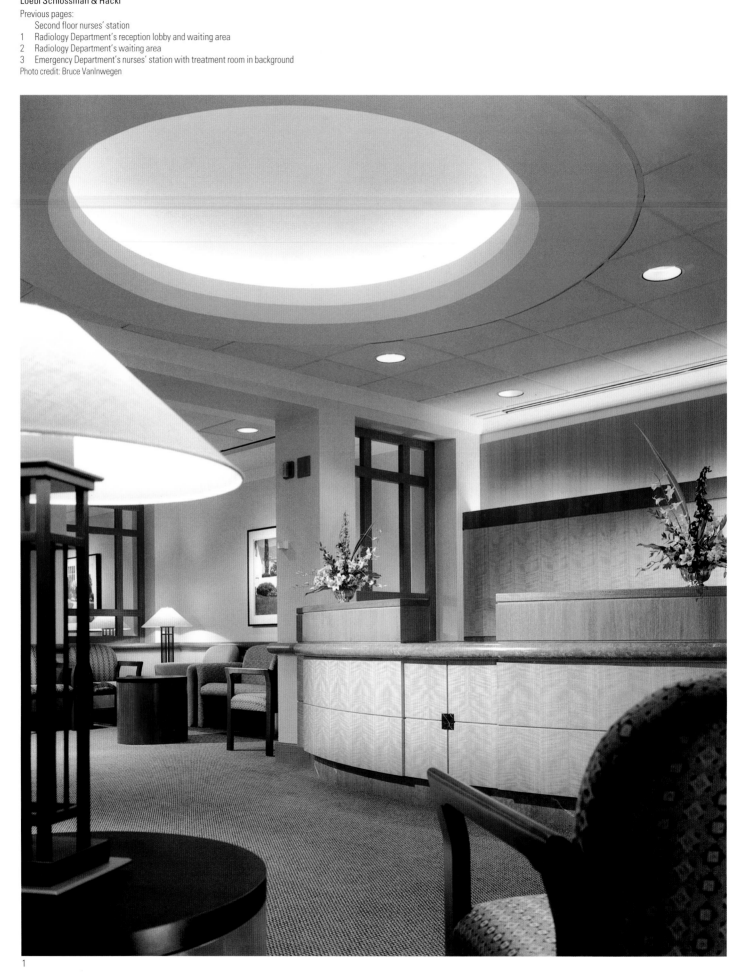

2

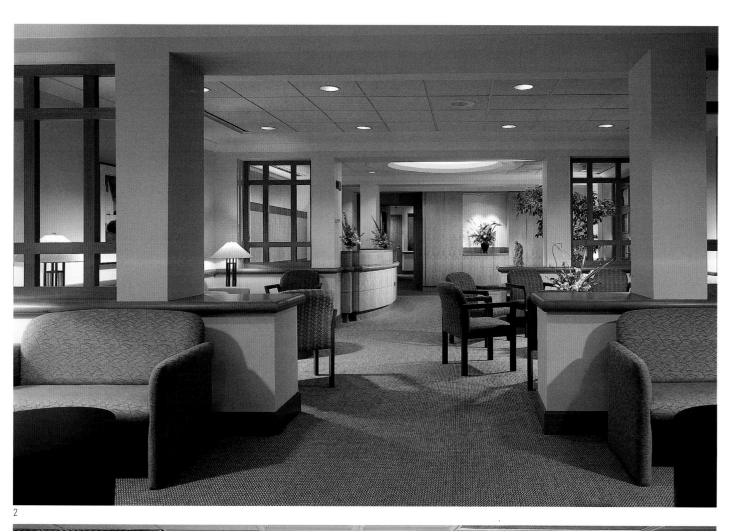

3

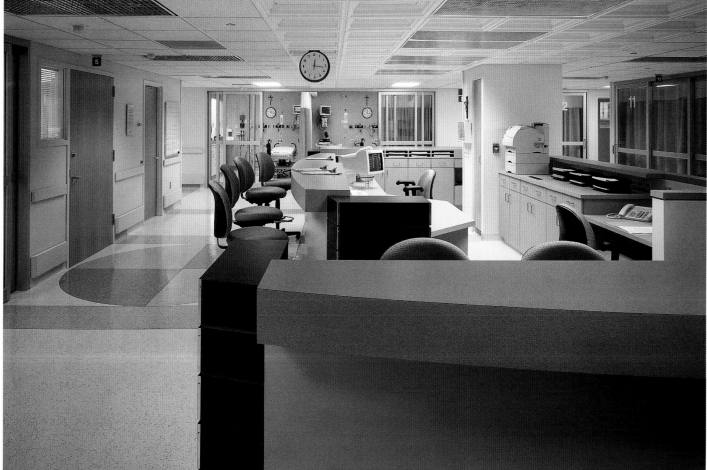

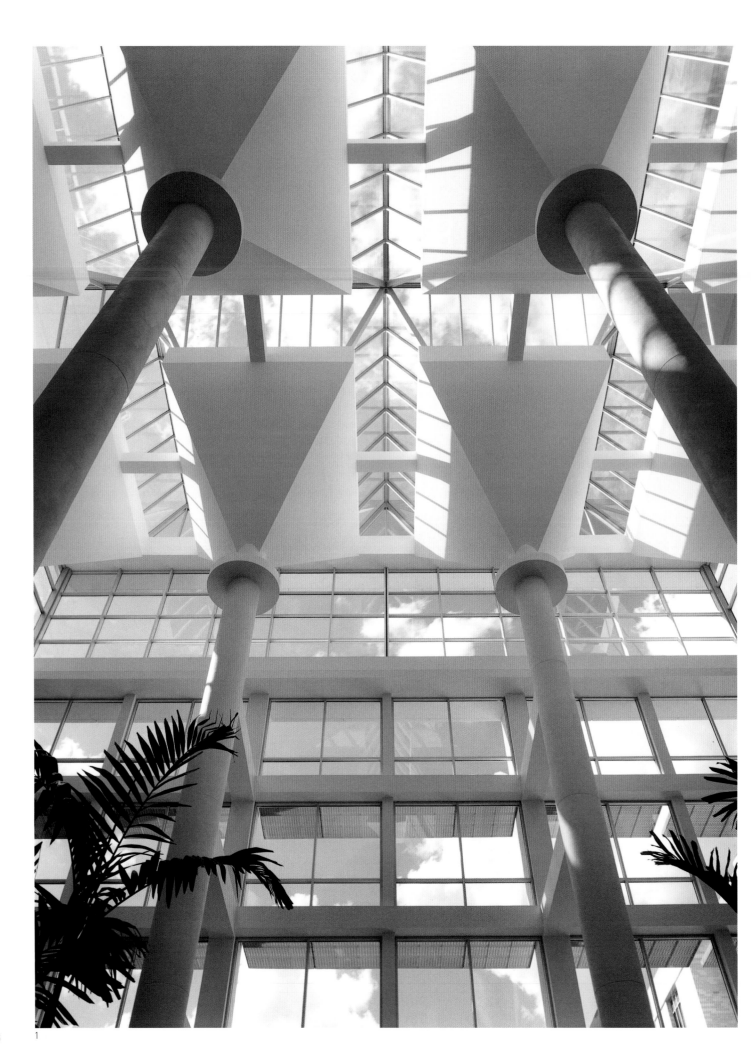

1

Good Samaritan Medical Center
West Palm Beach, Florida, USA
Payette Associates
1   Detail of atrium
2   Atrium
Photo credit: Brian Vanden Brink

University Center for Community Health
San Antonio, Texas, USA
Marmon Mok
3   Light filled generously proportioned circulation spine defies
    stigma of 'hospital corridor'
Photo credit: C. Blackmon

HealthPark Medical Center
Fort Myers, Florida, USA
HKS Inc.
4   CT scanner
5   Cardiac Cathiterisation Room
Photo credit: Rick Grumbaum

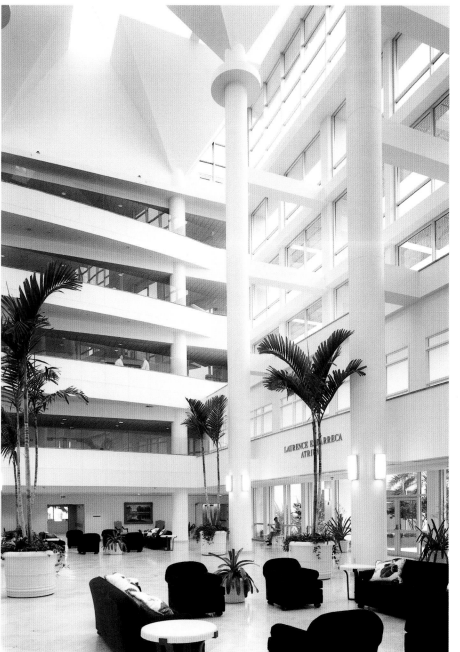

2

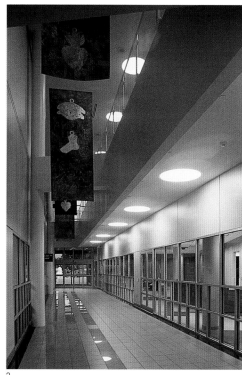

3

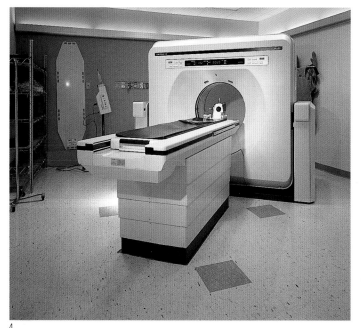

4

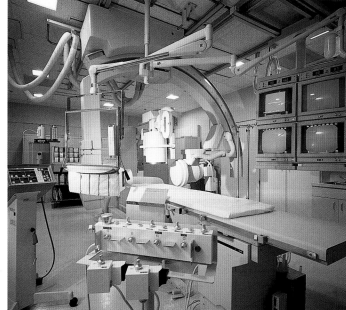

5

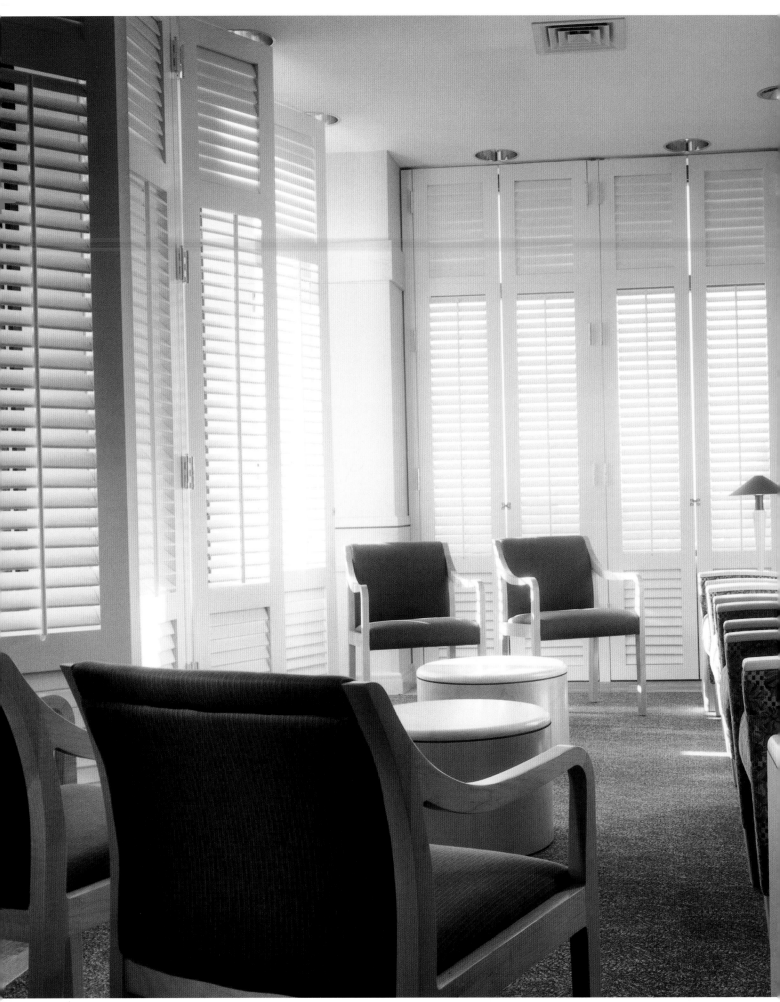

1

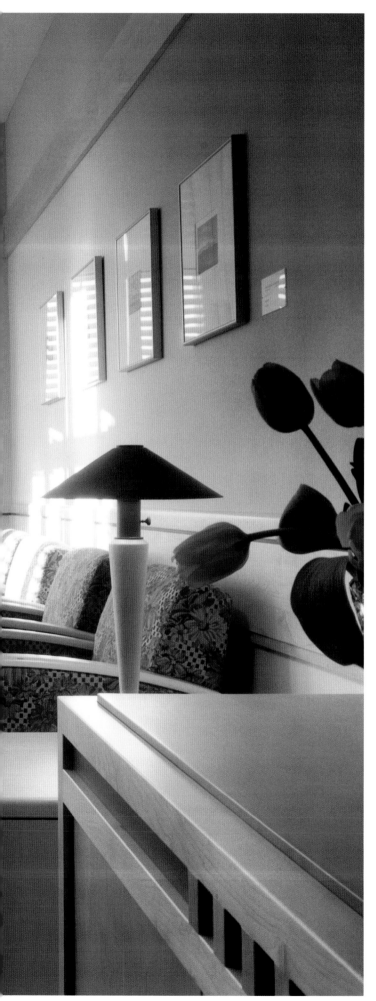

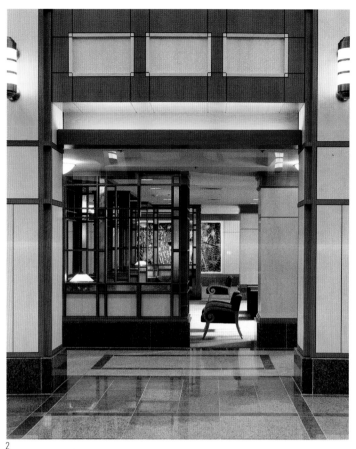

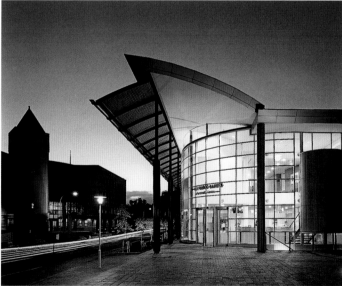

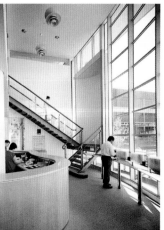

University Hospital of Cleveland, Alfred & Norma Lerner/Samuel Mather Pavilion
Cleveland, Ohio, USA
Payette Associates

1 Family waiting area/resting area for patients and staff
2 Visitor waiting area and patient solarium
Photo credit: Dan Forer

Blood Bank and Laboratories
Parramatta, NSW, Australia
Ancher Mortlock and Woolley

3 Exterior of reception area at dusk
4 Reception area
Photo credits: Eric Sierins (4); Eric Sierins/Max Dupain & Associates (3)

4

Greater Baltimore Medical Center
Baltimore, Maryland, USA
Loebl Schlossman & Hackl
1   Weinberg Community Health Center,
     reception and waiting area corridor
Photo credit: Alan Karchmer Photography

Aix en Provence Hospital
Aix en Provence, France
BDP Groupe 6
2   Exterior view to main entrance hall and
     waiting area
3   Interior view to main entrance hall and
     waiting area
Photo credit: courtesy of BDP Groupe 6

Edward Health and Fitness Center
at Seven Bridges
Woodridge, Illinois, USA
Phillips Swager Associates
4   Front desk at entry
5   Lobby area
Photo credit: Barry Rustin Photography

Swedish Medical Center
Seattle, Washington, USA
NBBJ
6   Main lobby rotunda for new addition
7   Ambulatory Care Center's waiting area
8   Pediatric wing area is scaled to a
     child's proportion
Photo credit: Steve Keating

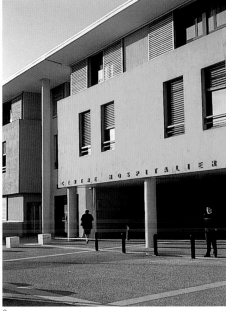
2

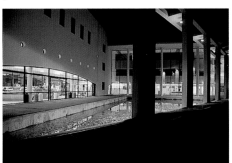
3

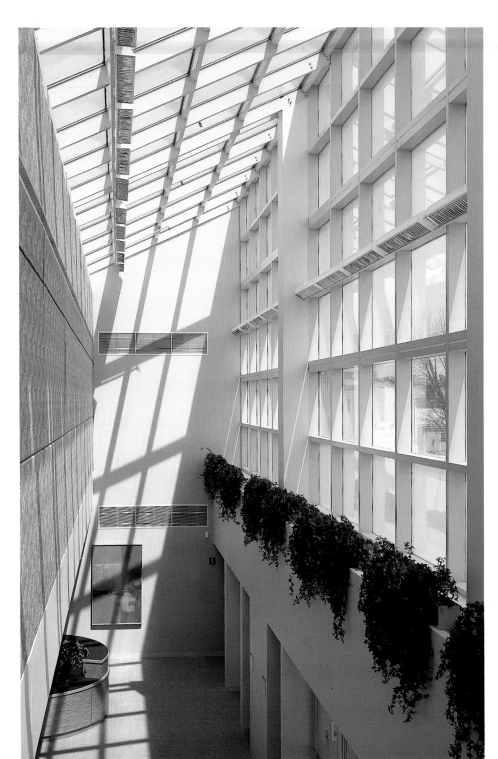

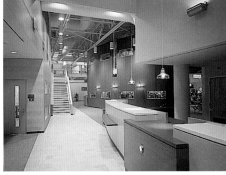

5

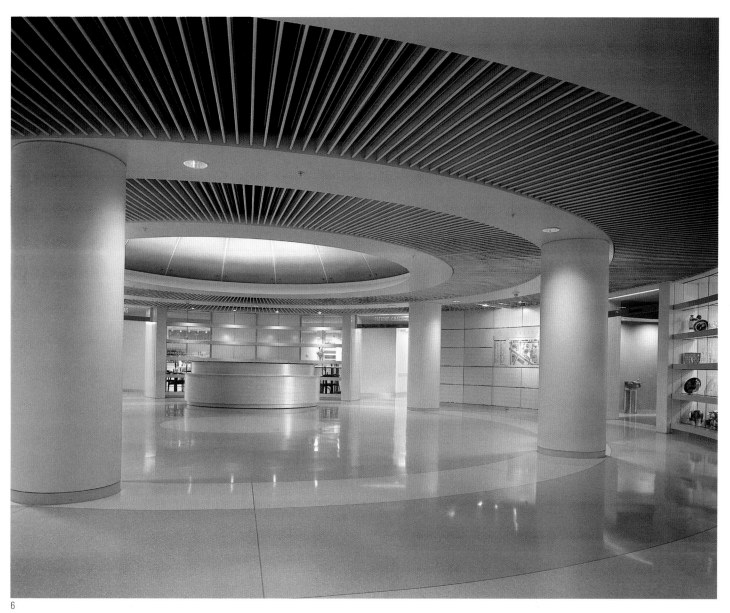

6

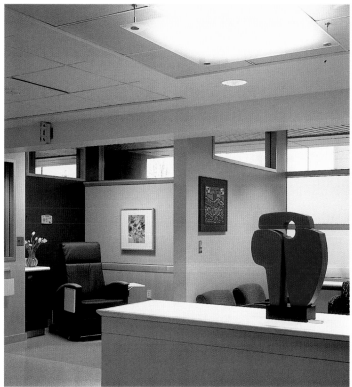

7

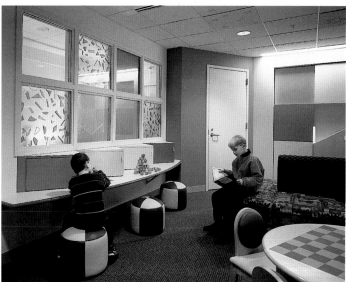

8

Swedish Medical Center
Seattle, Washington, USA
NBBJ

1   Ambulatory Care Center's waiting area
Photo credit: Steve Keating

HealthPark Medical Center
Fort Myers, Florida, USA
HKS Inc.

2   Atrium incorporates natural setting with
     tropical trees and vegetation
3   Atrium view from waiting area
4   View of atrium and foyer
5   Atrium from balcony view
Photo credit: Rick Grumbaum

Gottlieb Memorial Hospital
Melrose Park, Illinois, USA
Loebl Schlossman & Hackl

Opposite bottom:
     Marjorie G. Weinberg Cancer Care Center,
     reception and waiting area
Photo credit: James Steinkamp,
Stienkamp/Ballogg Photography

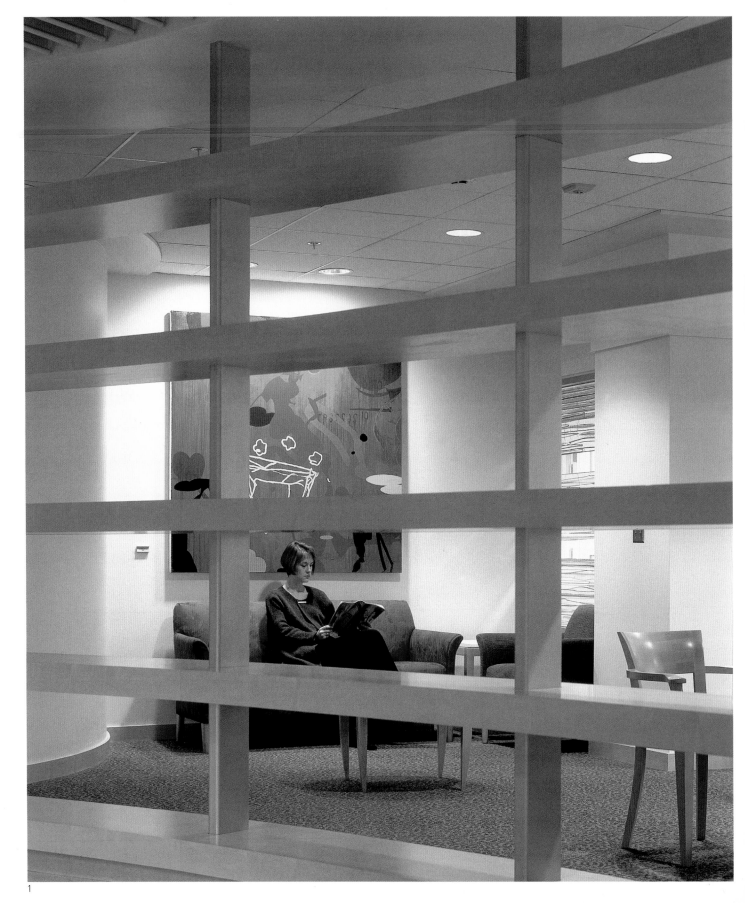

1

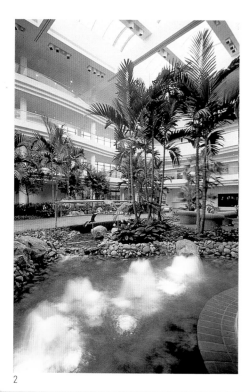

2

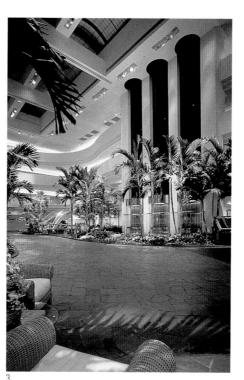

3

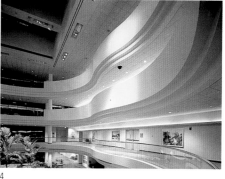

4

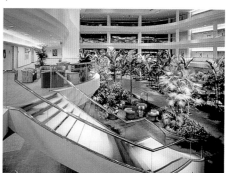

5

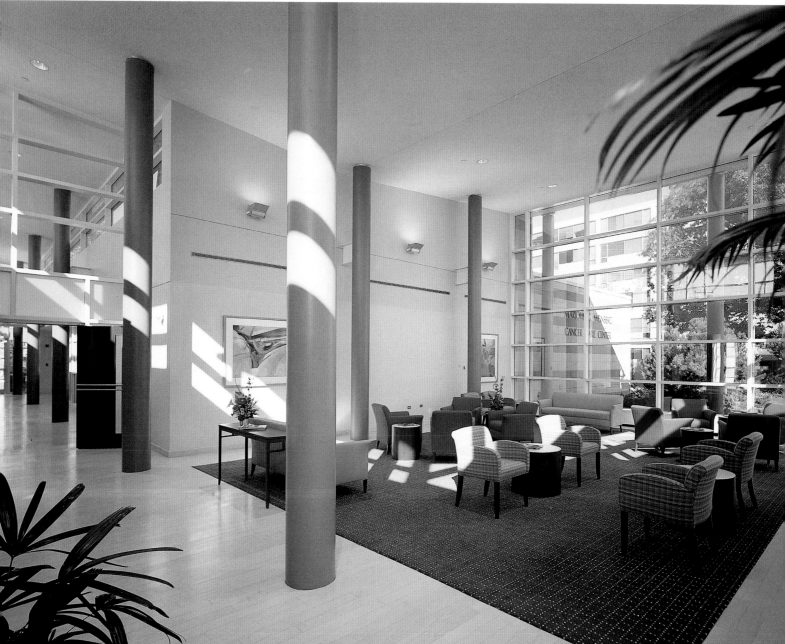

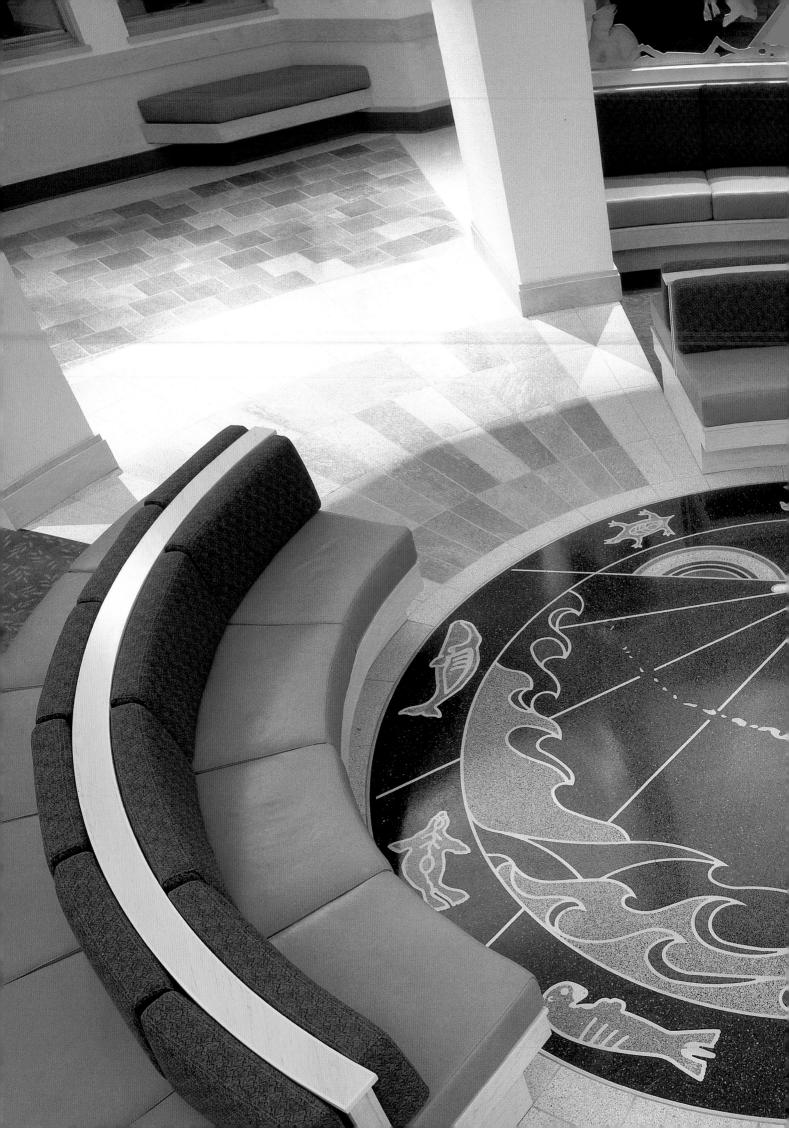

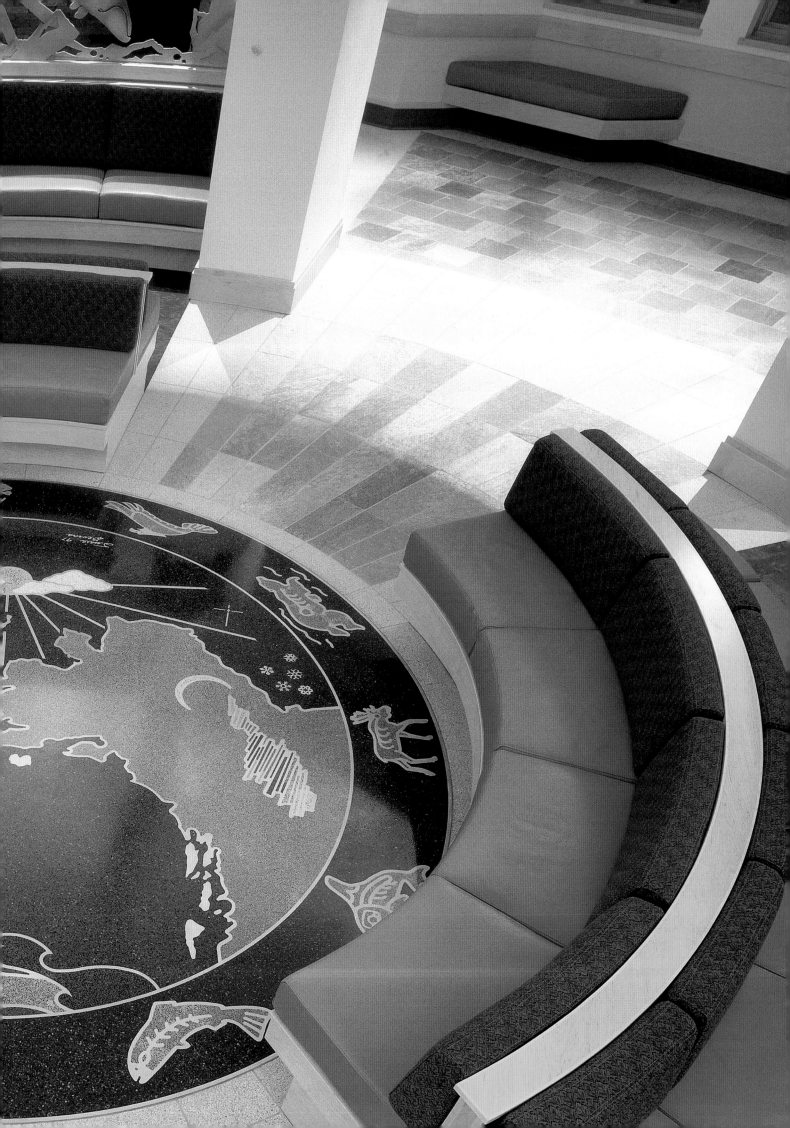

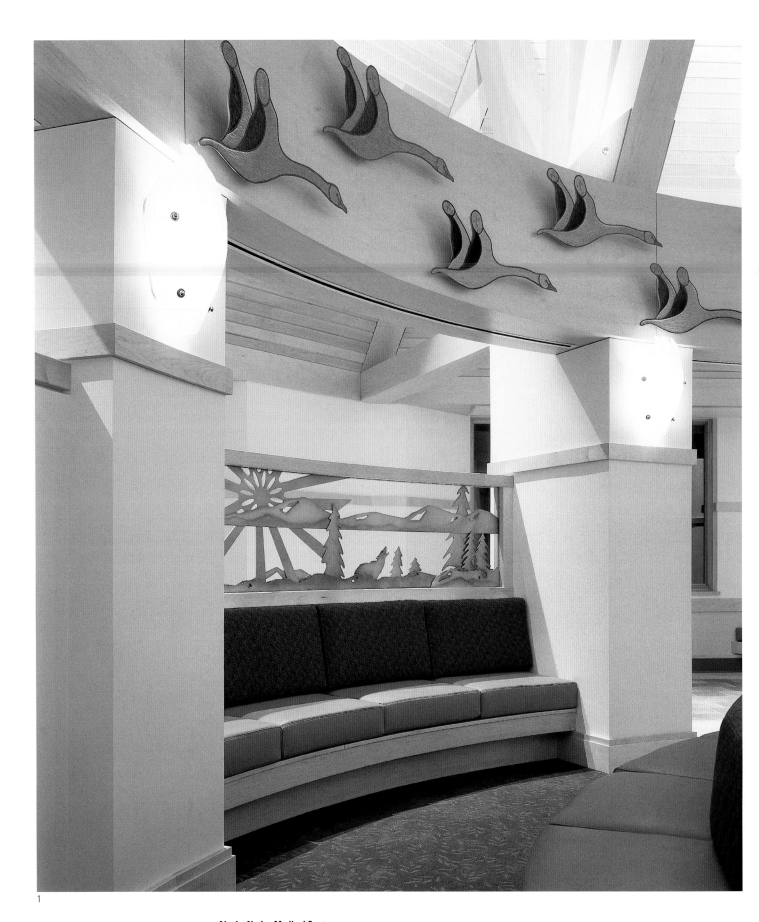

1

Alaska Native Medical Center
Anchorage, Alaska, USA
NBBJ

Previous pages:
    Spirit House and lobby terrazzo floor
1   Art in main lobby reflecting Alaskan region
Opposite:
    Main waiting and lobby area at Spirit House
Photo credit: Assassi Productions

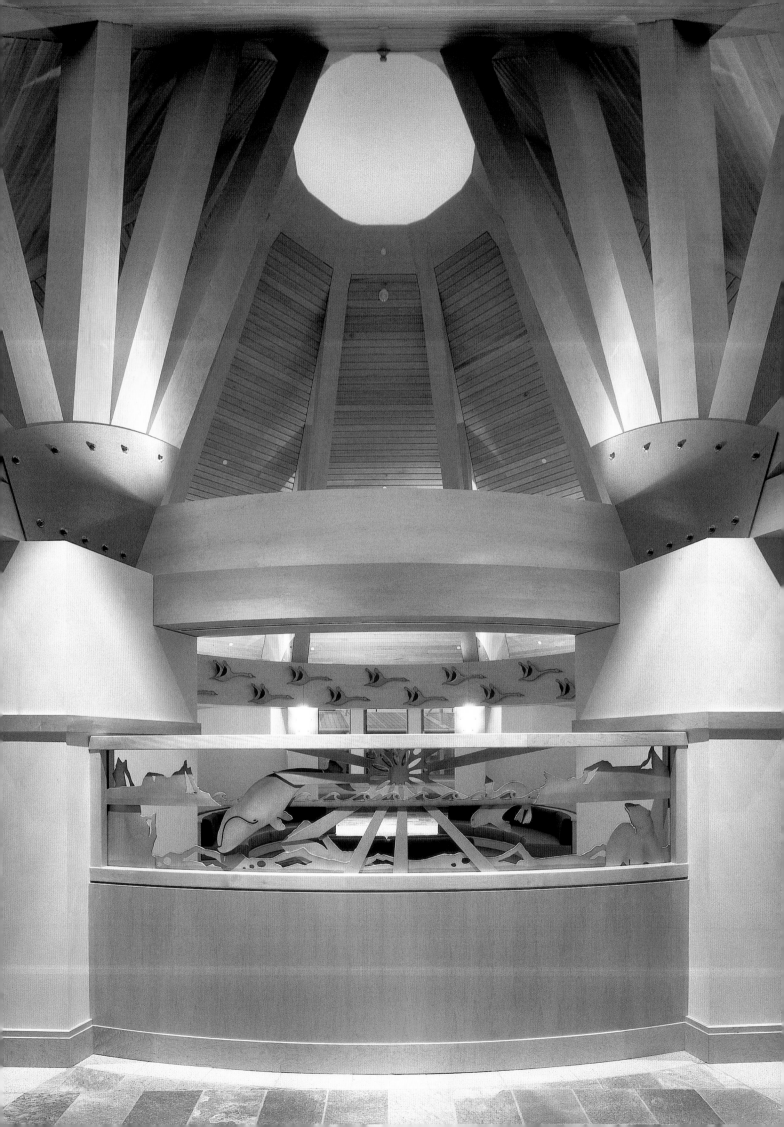

Ontario Cancer Institute–Princess
Margaret Hospital
Toronto, Canada
Hellmuth, Obata + Kassabaum, Inc.
1   Reception area
Photo credit: courtesy of Hellmuth, Obata
+ Kassabaum, Inc.

Alaska Native Medical Center
Anchorage, Alaska, USA
NBBJ
2   Expansive views create meditative spaces
      for patient relaxation
3   Main corridor
Photo credit: Paul Warchol (2);
Assassi Productions (3)

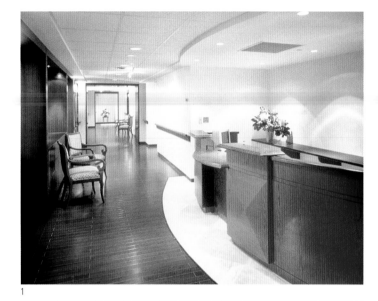

1

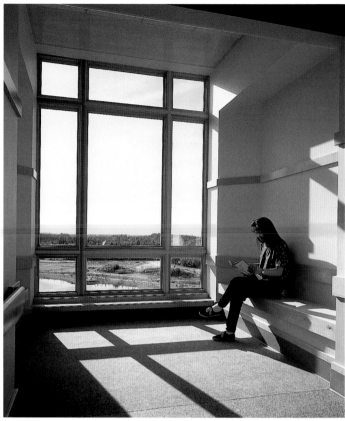

2

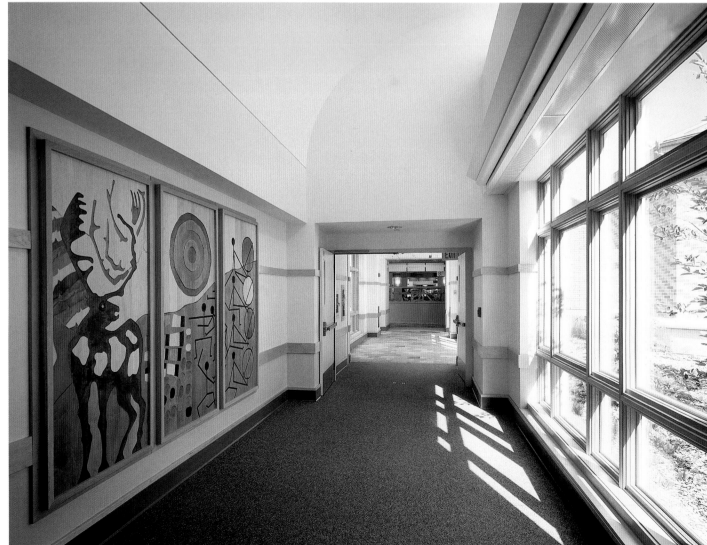

3

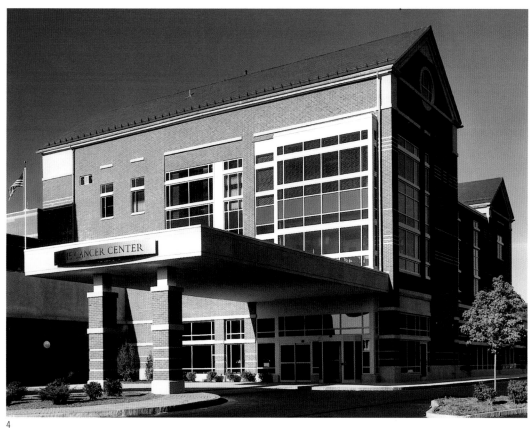

Lowell General Hospital,
Cancer Care Center
Lowell, Massachusetts, USA
TRO/The Ritchie Organization
4   Front façade
Below:
    Patients and families are welcomed at
    reception with uplifting messages and a
    palette of warm colours and natural
    materials
Following pages:
    Open area is sculpted by light and
    architecture to reinforce zones of use
Photo credit: Edward Jacoby/Jacoby Photography

4

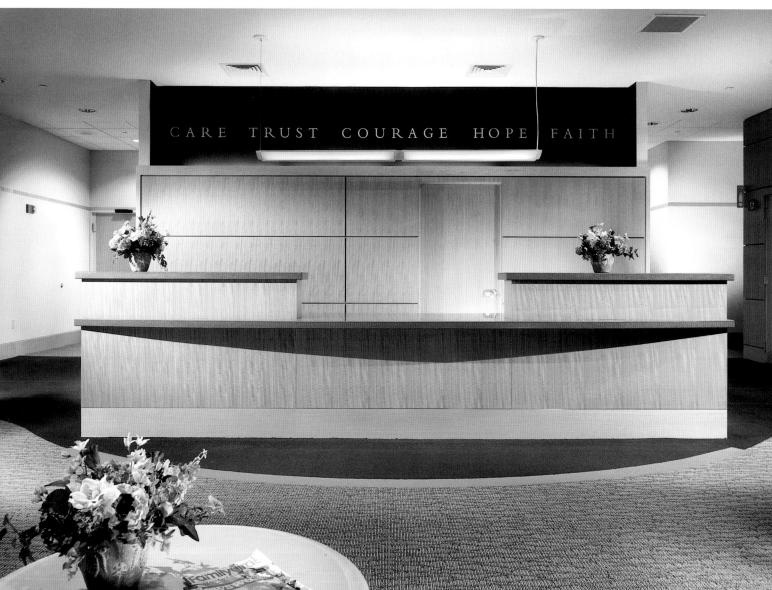

CARE   TRUST   COURAGE   HOPE   FAITH

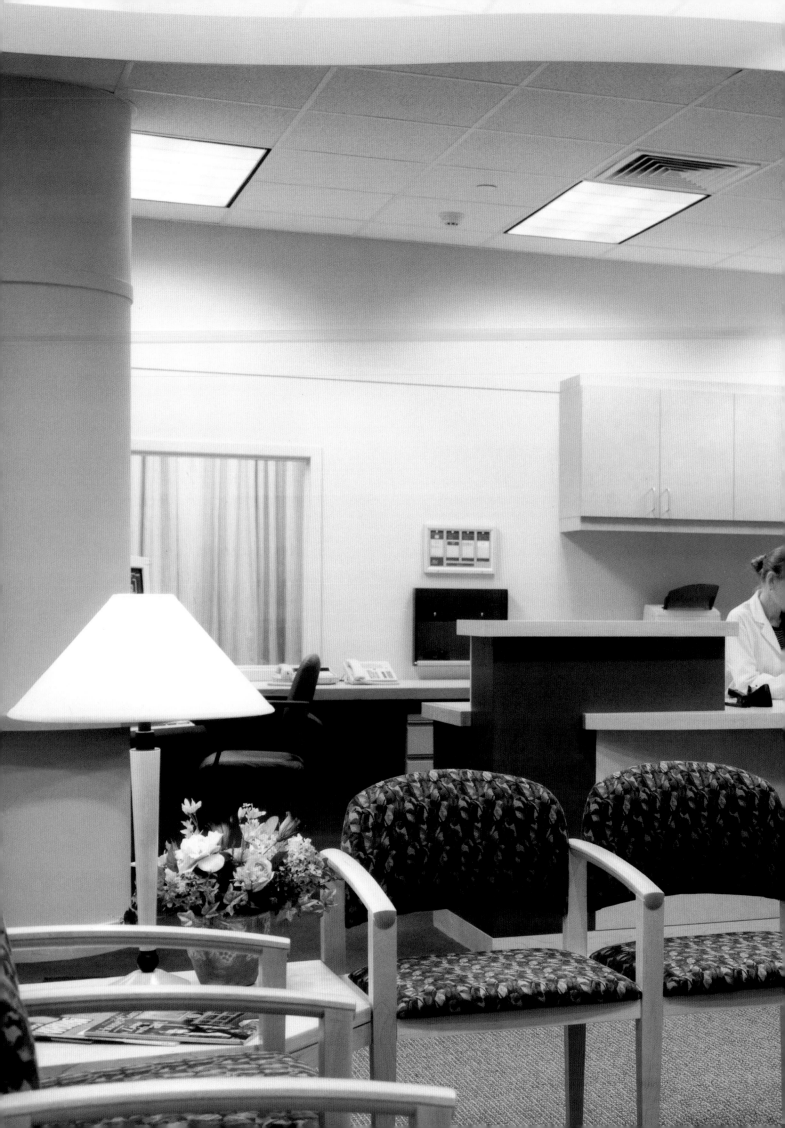

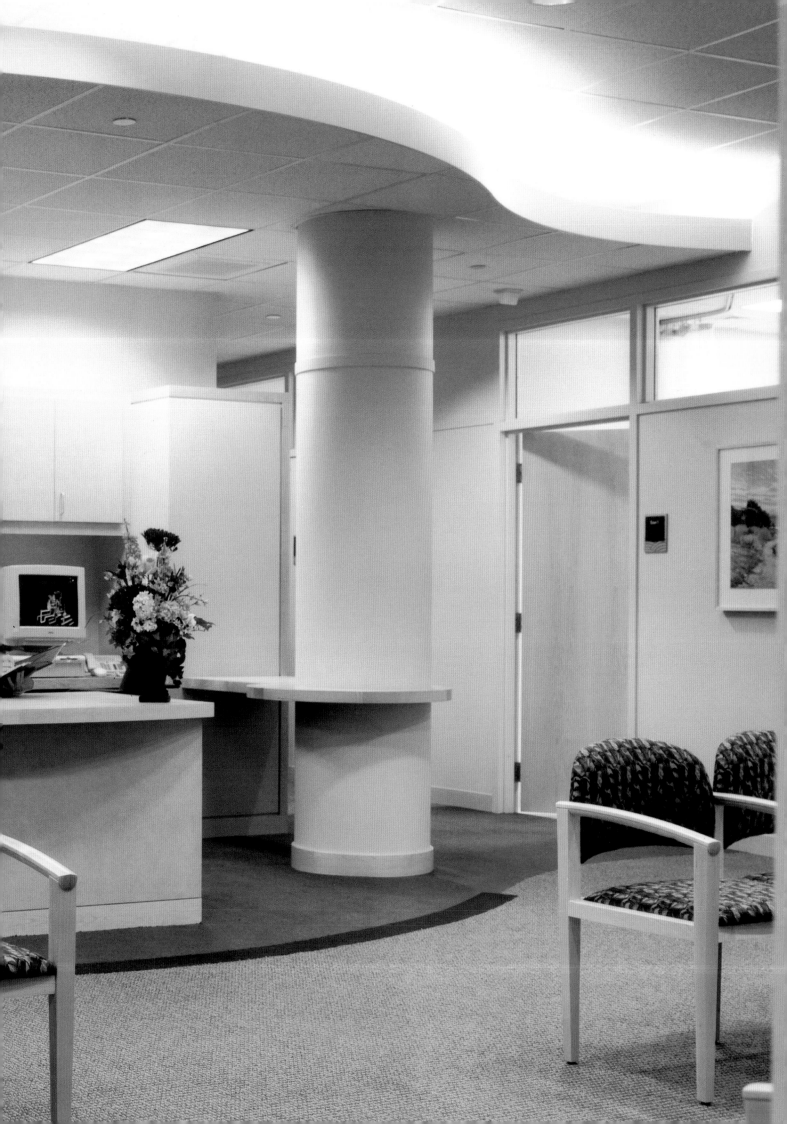

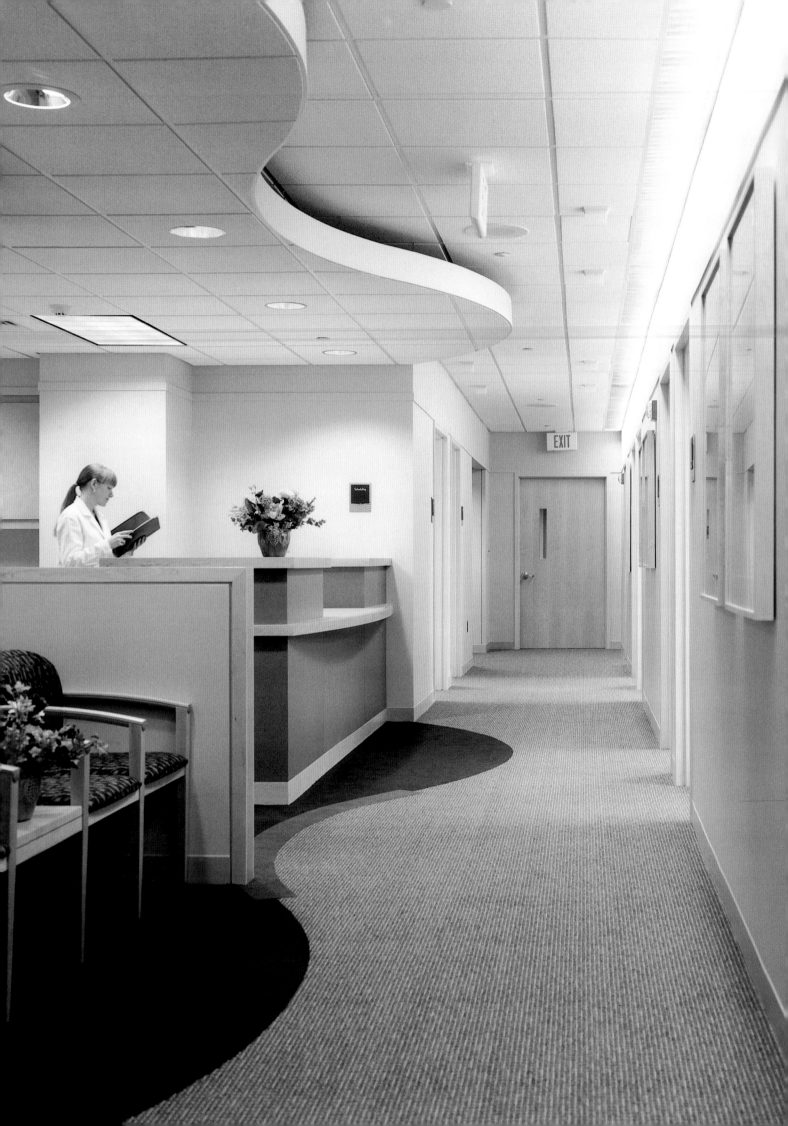

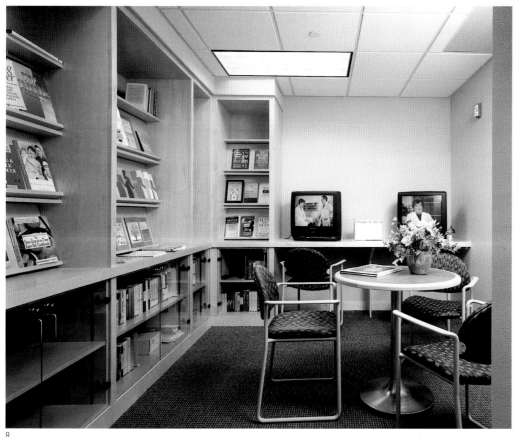

**Lowell General Hospital,
Cancer Care Center
Lowell, Massachusetts, USA**
TRO/The Ritchie Organization
Opposite:
      Carpet patterns and natural lighting
      guides patients to nurses' station and
      waiting areas
8&9   Reading and waiting area
Following pages:
      Main lobby is filled with natural light
      and soothing sounds from aquarium
Photo credit: Edward Jacoby/Jacoby Photography

8

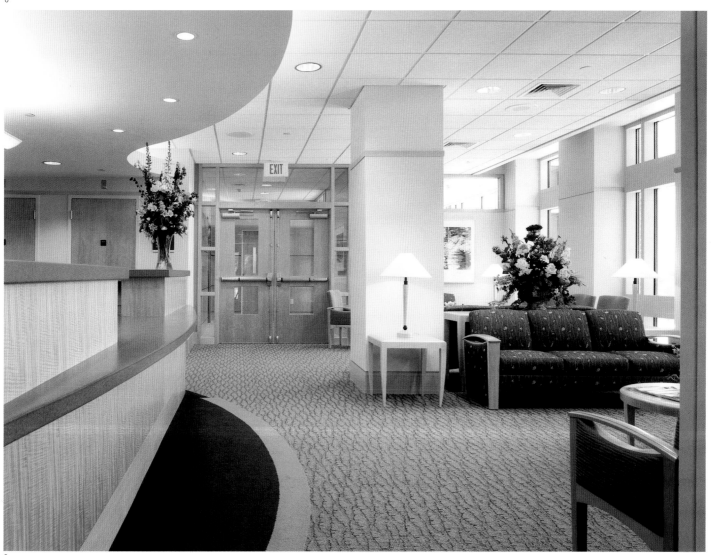

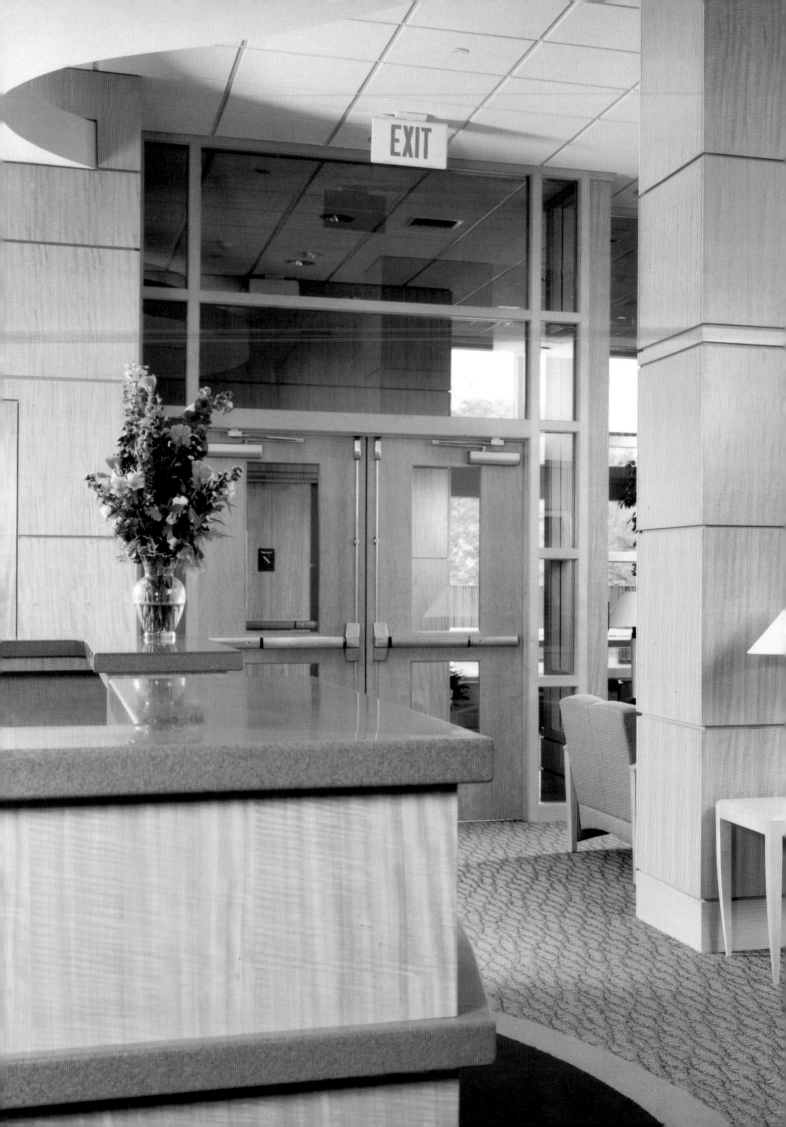

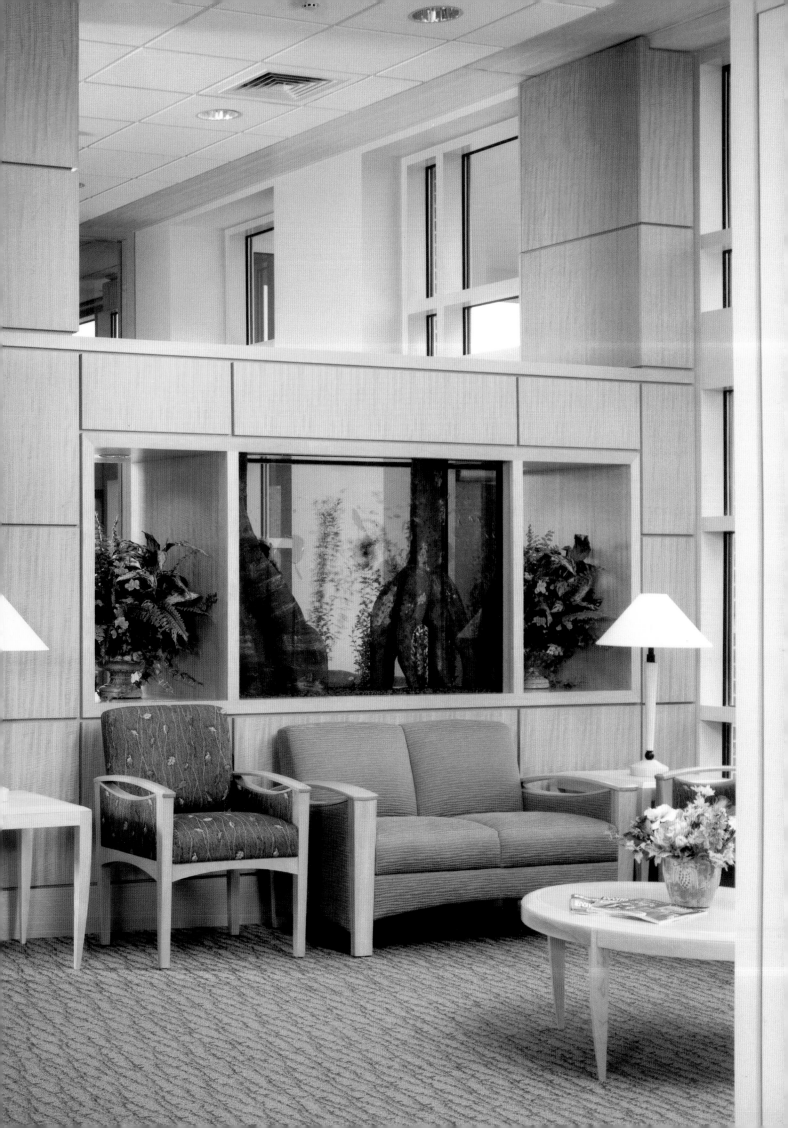

Northeast Georgia Health Services–Short Stay Surgery
Gainsville, Georgia, USA
Quantrell Mullins & Associates Inc.

1 Reception area
2 Waiting area
3 Vending area
4 Children's play/waiting area
Photo credit: Brian Robbins

The National Children's Center
Anacostia, Washington, D.C., USA
CUH2A

5 Reception area introduces visitors to light filled, airy and commodious interior space
6 Interior street filled with skylights and opening onto both enclosed and exterior courtyards
7 Building is designed like a toy construction kit, resulting in instructive and playful spaces
Photo credit: Ron Blunt

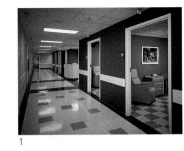
1

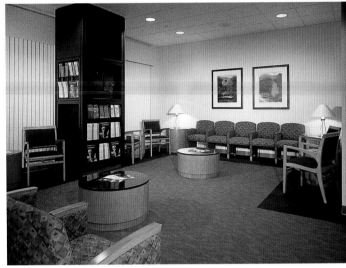
2

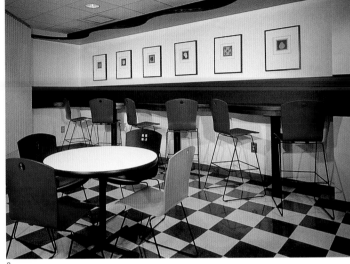
3

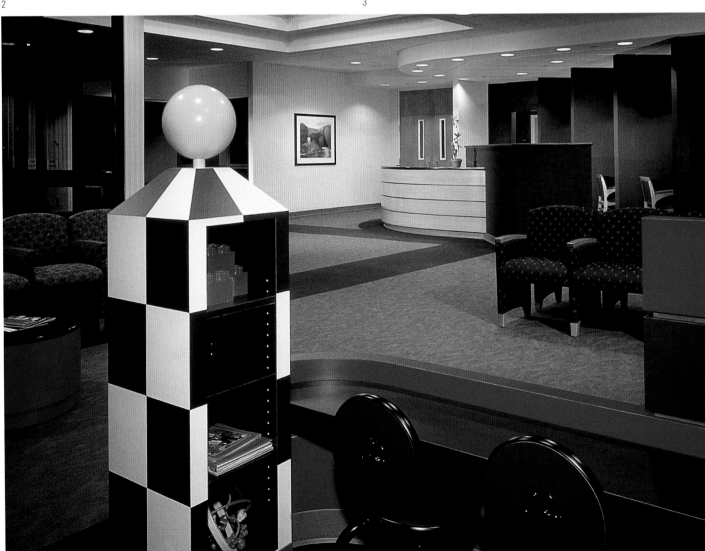

4

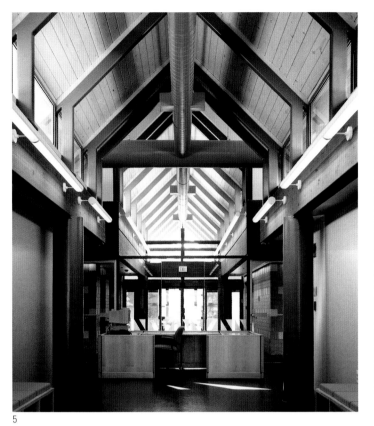

5

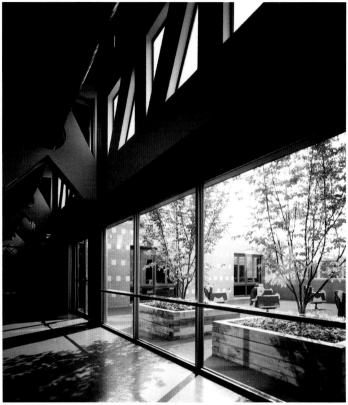

6

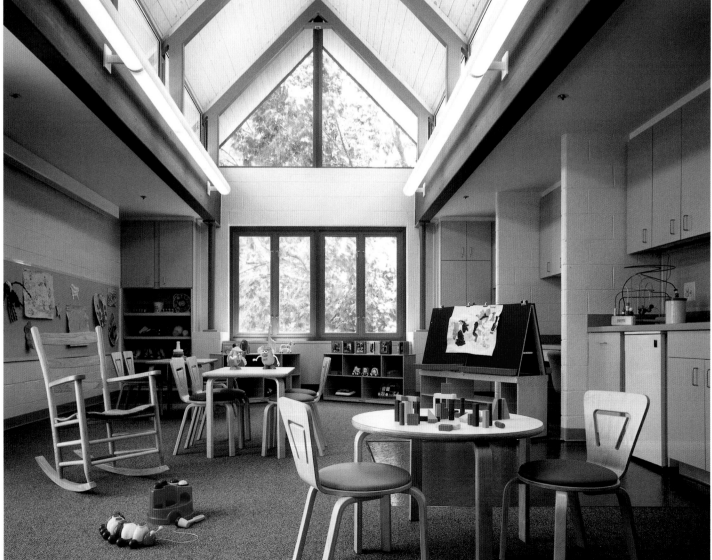

7

Aikman's End Zone, Cook Children's Fort Worth Hospital
Fort Worth, Texas, USA
HKS Inc.

1   Entrance with two aquariums
2   'Starbright', interactive computers
3   Eight-foot replica of Aikman's helmet
4   Donor wall
Photo credit: Ron St. Angelo

Dublin Dental Hospital,
Refurbishment and New Wing
Trinity College, Dublin, Ireland
Ahrends Burton and Koralek

5   Old building and extension on Lincoln Place
Photo credit: Peter Cook/VIEW

Scottsdale Memorial Hospital
North Pavilion
Scottsdale, Arizona, USA
NBBJ

6   View from northeast
7   Entry court
Photo credit: Peter Aaron/Esto

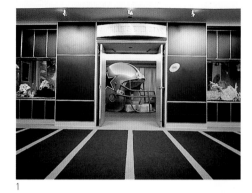

1

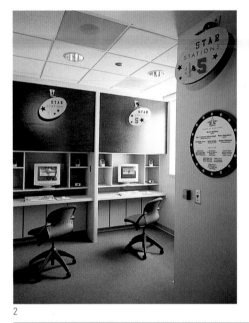

2

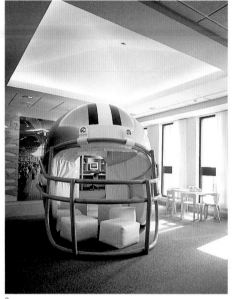

3

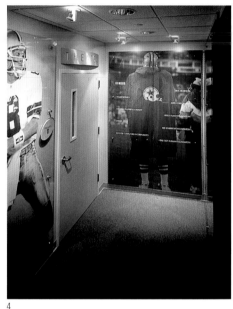

4

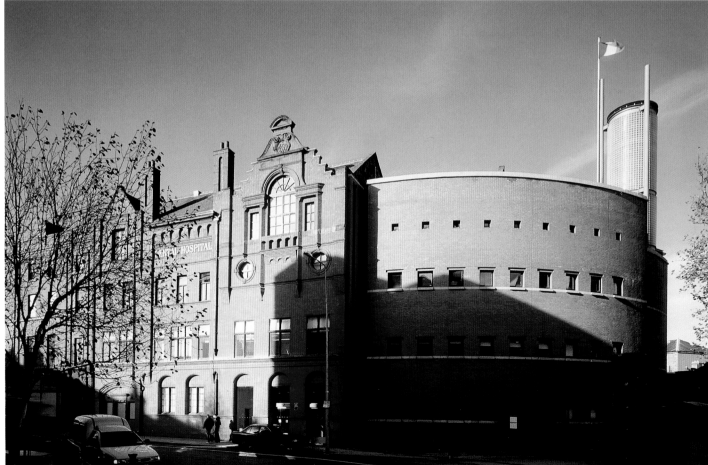

5

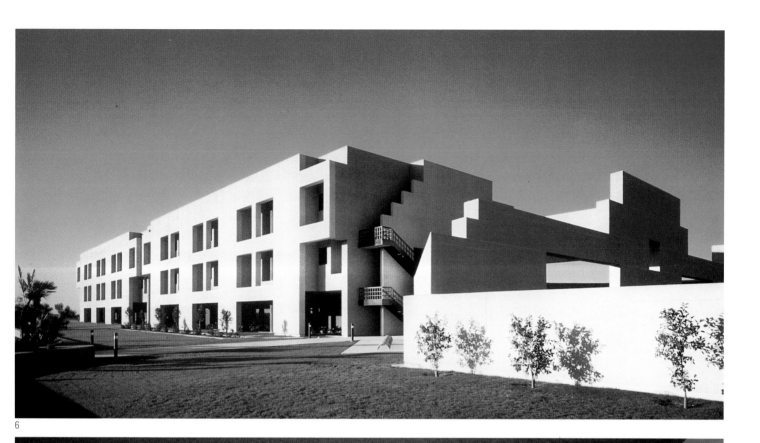

6

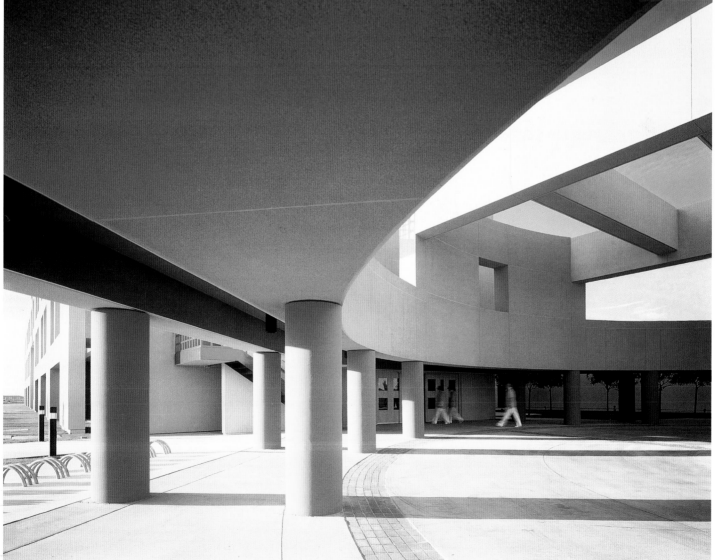

WestHealth
Minneapolis, Minnesota, USA
Ellerbe Becket, Inc.

1   Same day surgery waiting area
2   Public elevator lobby
3   Same day surgery patient care suites
4   Same day surgery
5   Main lobby/atrium
Photo credit: Koyama Photographic

Phoebe Northwest, Phoebe Putney
Memorial Hospital
Albany, Georgia, USA
TRO/The Ritchie Organization

6   Family Care Centre waiting area
7   Main reception and waiting area
Photo credit: George Cott

Central Washington Hospital,
Additions & Alterations
Wenatchee, Washington, USA
NBBJ

Opposite:
    Surgery rotunda at control desk
Photo credit: Paul Warchol

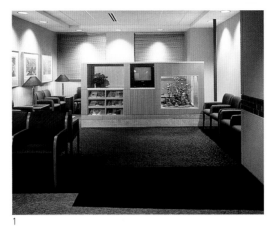
1

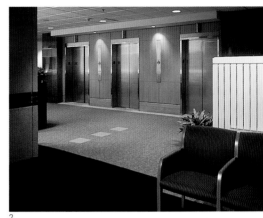
2

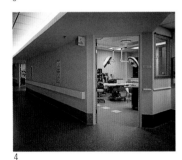
3

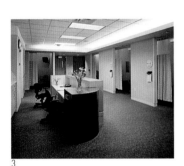
4

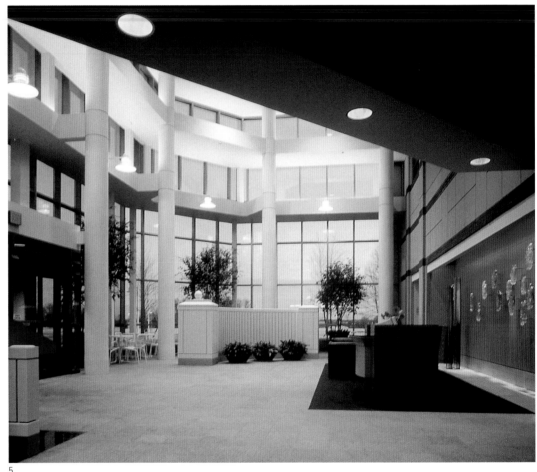
5

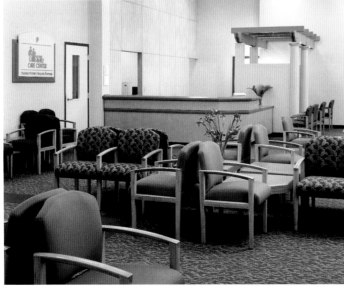
6

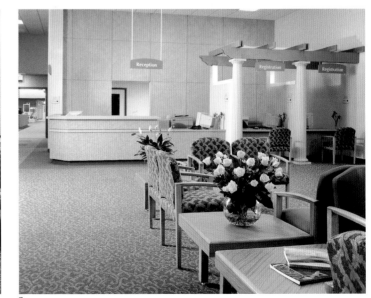
7

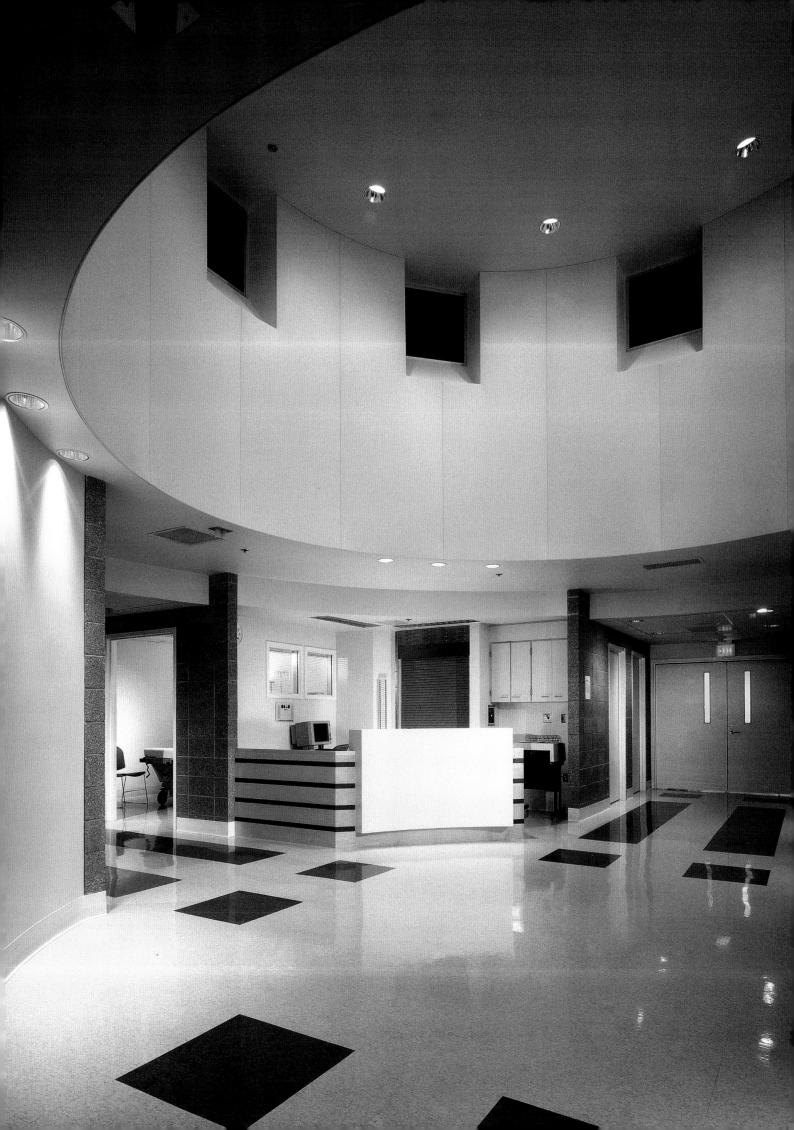

**Central Washington Hospital,
Additions & Alterations
Wenatchee, Washington, USA**
NBBJ
9   Ambulatory surgery wing entry arcade
10   Exterior view
Below:
     Corridor
12   Surgery entrance with Emergency
      Treatment Facility in left background
13   Waiting area
Photo credit: Paul Warchol

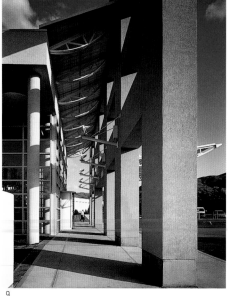

9

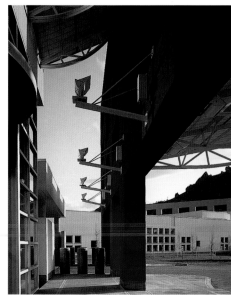

10

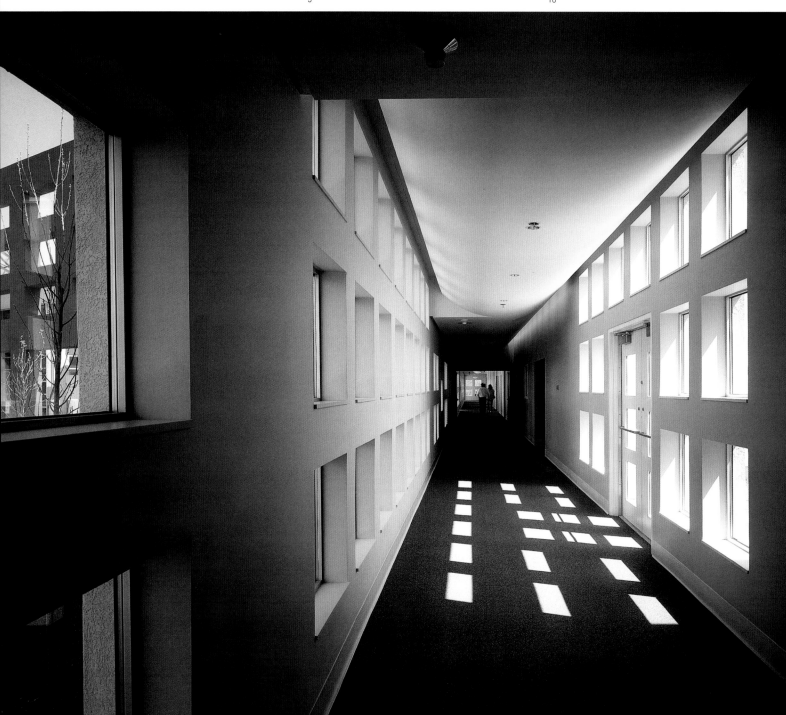

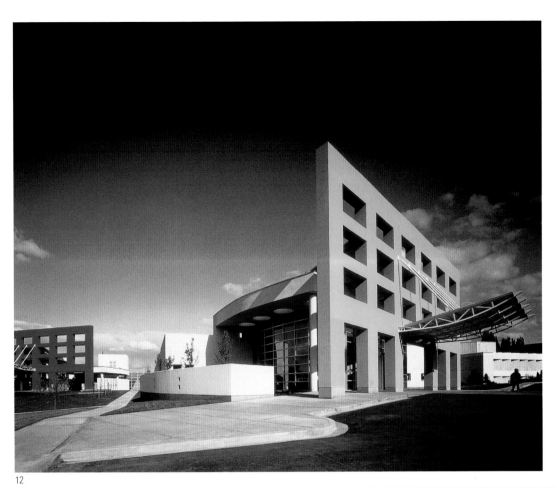

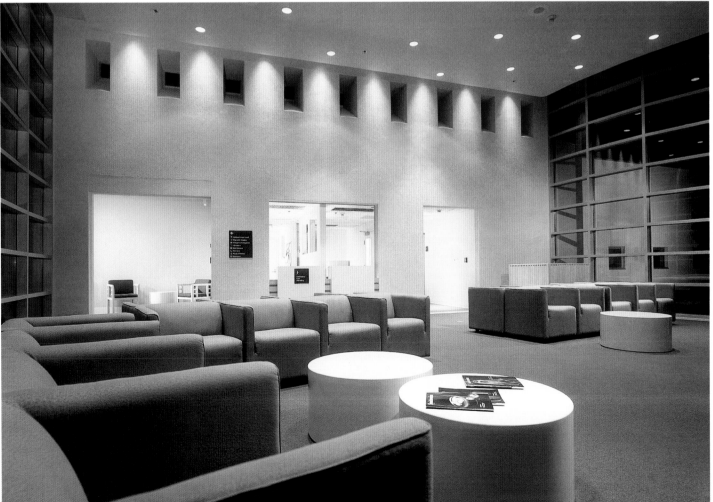

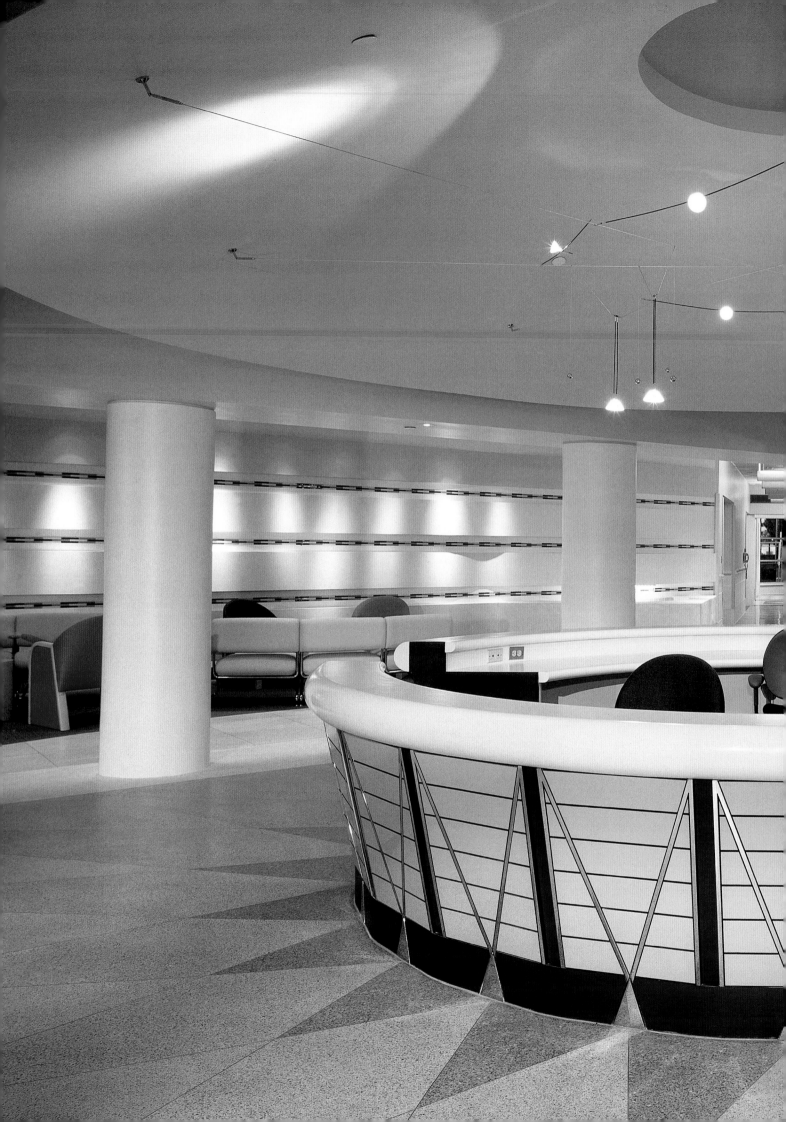

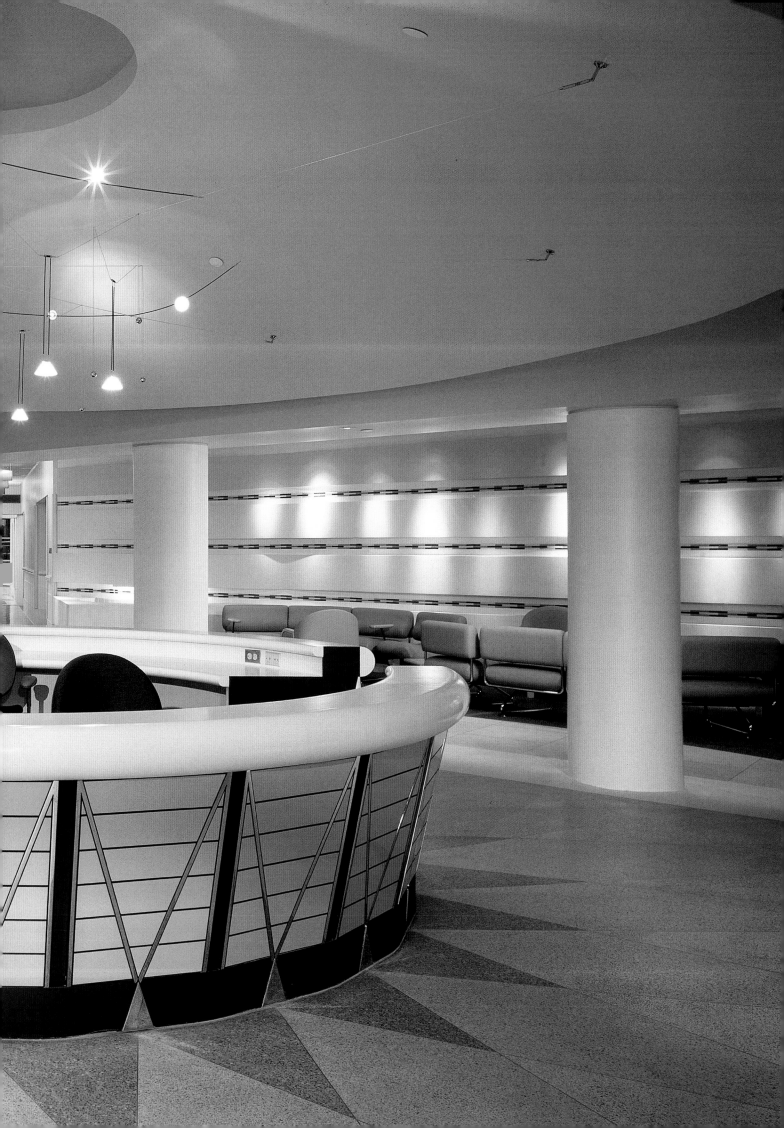

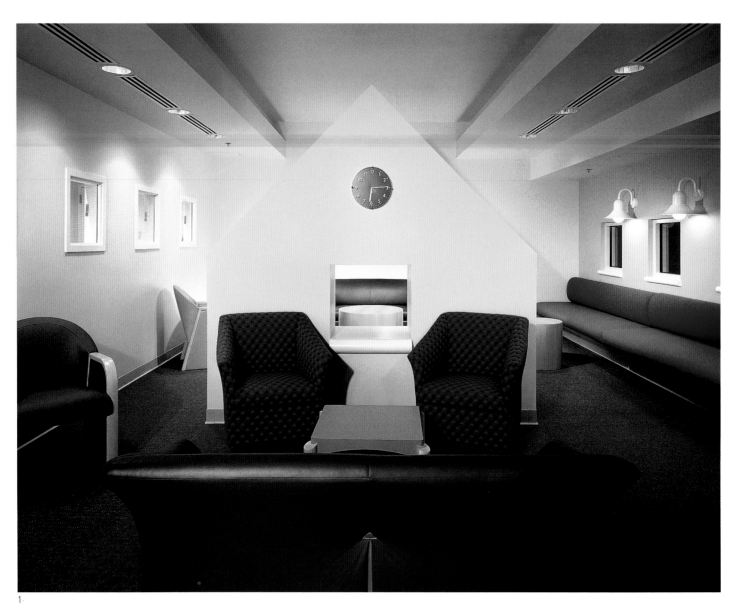

1

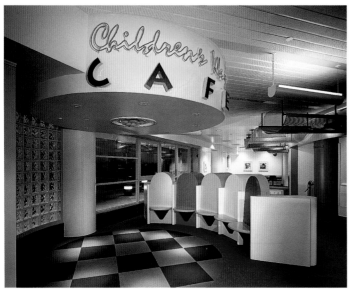

2

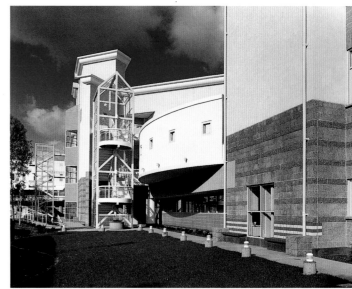

3

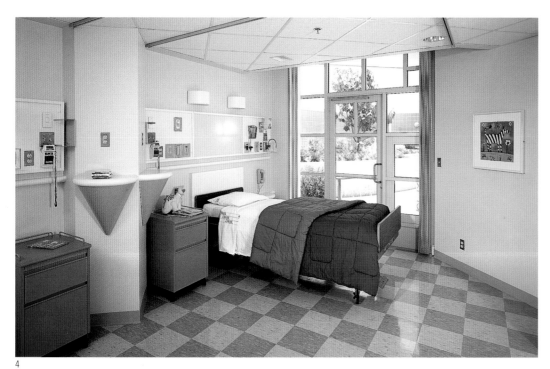

4

Children's Hospital and Health Center,
Patient Care Pavilion
San Diego, California, USA
NBBJ
Previous pages:
   Reception lobby
1   Family waiting room
2   Children's Way Café
3   Exterior stair and courtyard balcony
4   Double patient room
5   Nursing station with fibre-optic star field
   overhead
Photo credit: David Hewitt & Anne Garrison

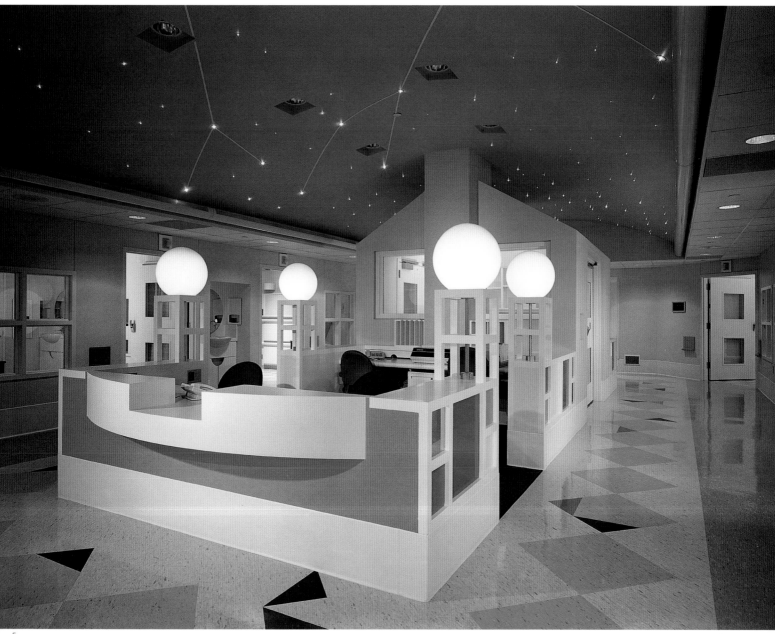

5

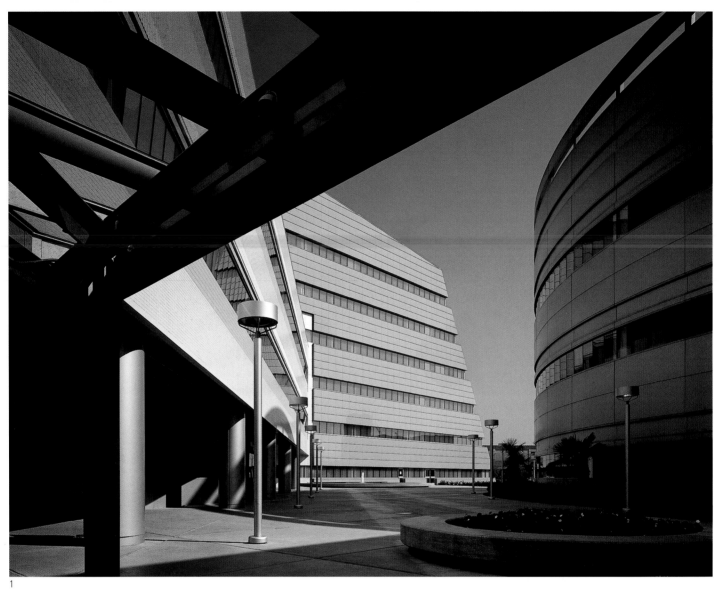

1

Baldwin Park Medical Center
Baldwin Park, California, USA
HMC Group with Arthur Erickson
& Associates

1   Patient/visitor drop-off and main entrance
2   Medical Center rotunda lobby
3   Interior corridor with daylight
4   View of park and lagoon with patient tower
    (green) and medical office building (silver)
    beyond
5   Roof garden
Following pages:
    Cafeteria dining area
Photo credit: courtesy of HMC Group with Arthur
Erickson & Associates

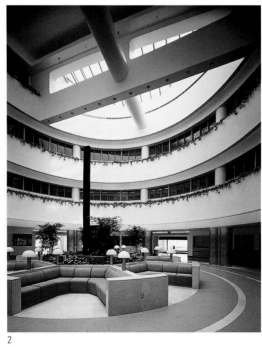

2

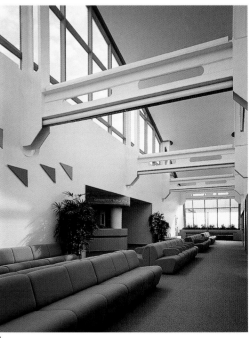

3

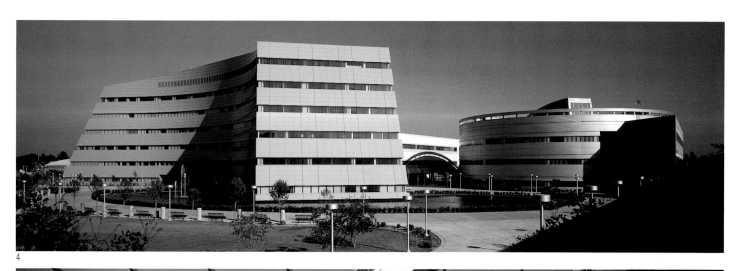

4

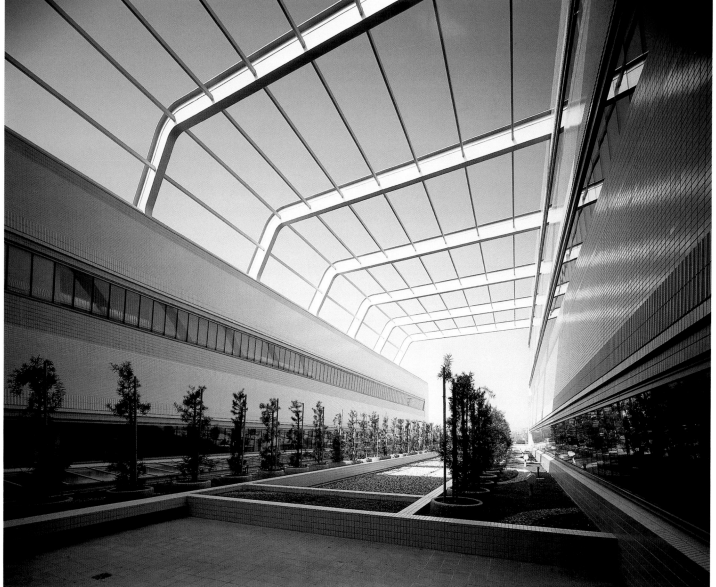

5

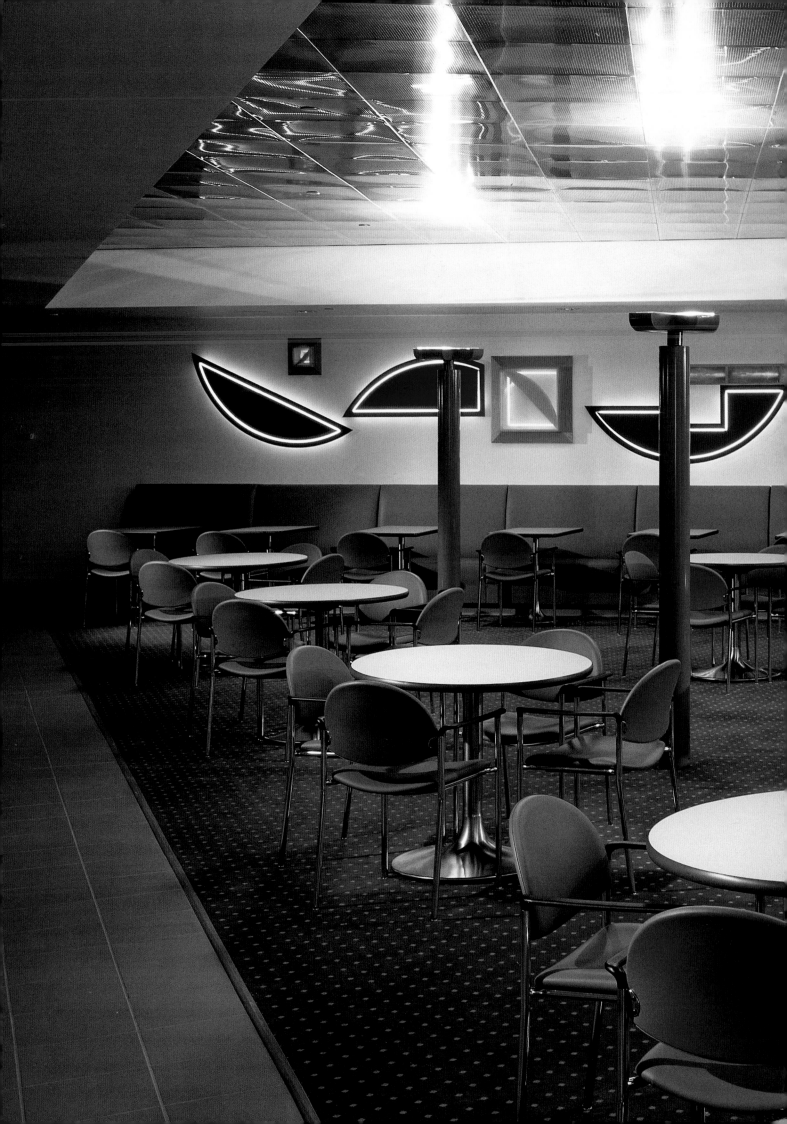

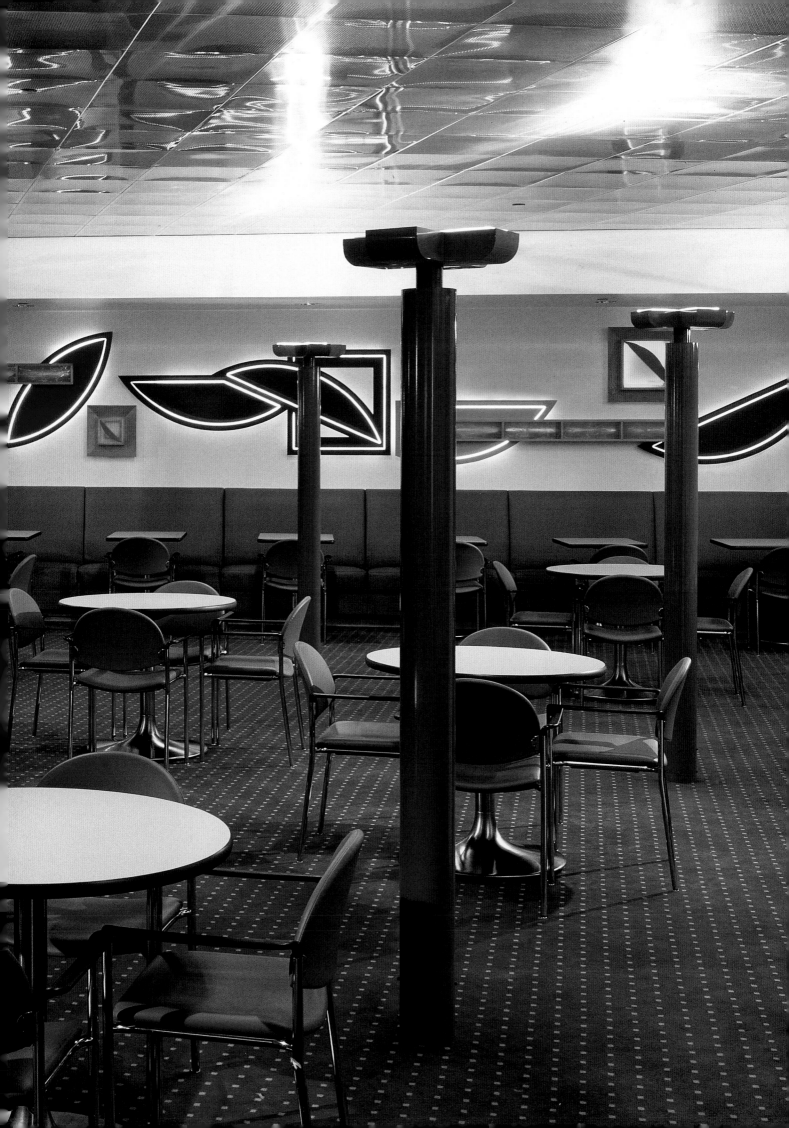

Milford Hospital, Patient Care Building
Milford, Connecticut, USA
TRO/The Ritchie Organization

1   Drop off area is covered for patient comfort
2   Medical gases are concealed within
    caseword in LDRP patient rooms
Opposite:
    Main lobby serves as comfortable waiting
    place as well as important wayfinding
    vehicle
Photo credit: Edward Jacoby/Jacoby Photography

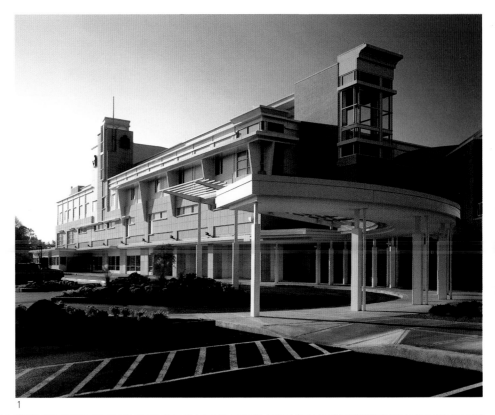

1

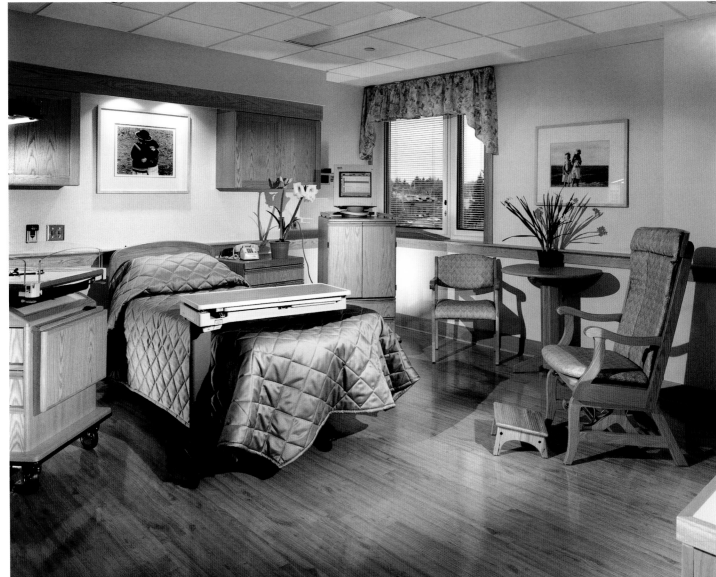

2

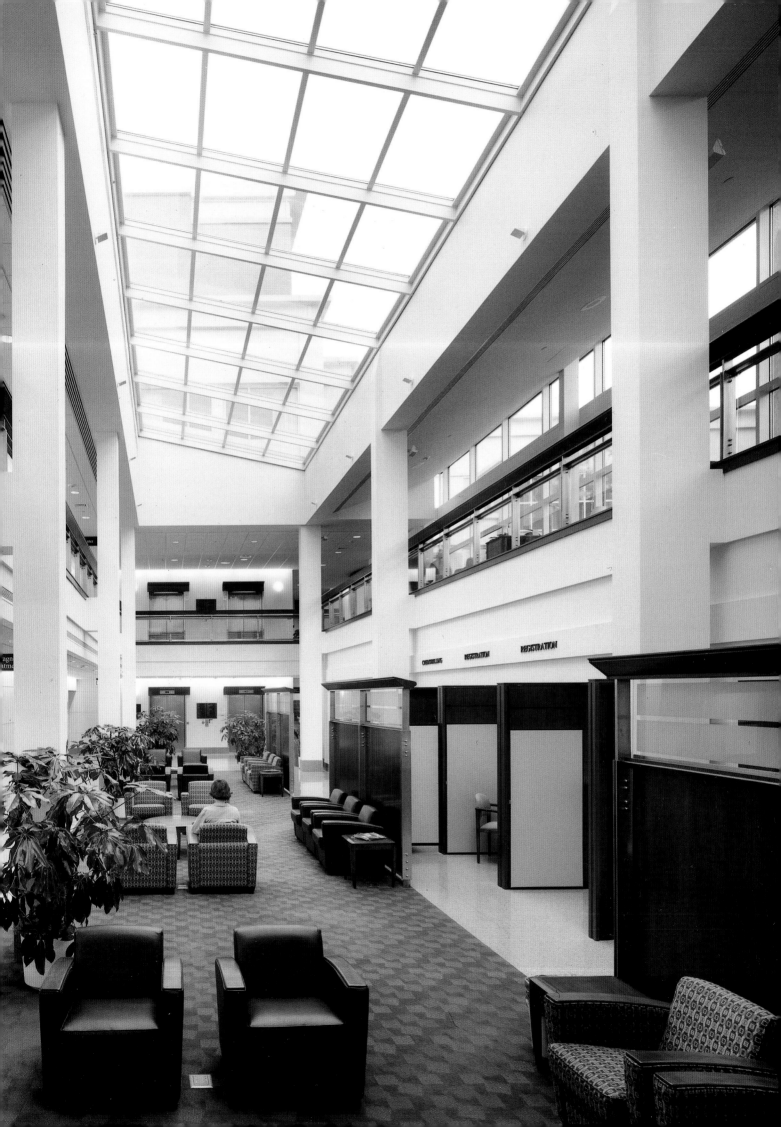

Toowoomba Hospital Redevelopment
Toowoomba, Qld, Australia
Bligh Nield Health

1   Resuscitation Bay
2   Intensive Care Unit with external windows
3   Medical Imaging Room
Photo credit: David Sandison

Milford Hospital Patient Care Building
Milford, Connecticut, USA
TRO/The Ritchie Organization

4   Oversized intensive care unit rooms were
    well planned to facilitate all medical
    scenarios
Photo credit: Edward Jacoby/Jacoby Photography

SEASONS: A Center for Renewal
Kalamazoo, Michigan, USA
HarleyEllis

5   Interior with vaulted roof structure
Photo credit: Gay Quesada/Hedrich-Blessing

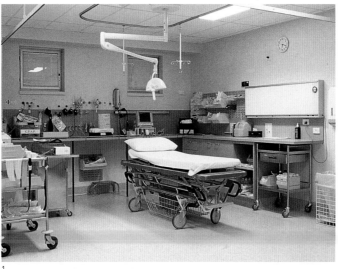

1

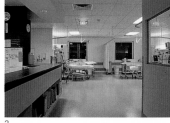

2

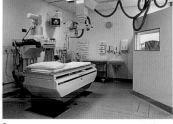

3

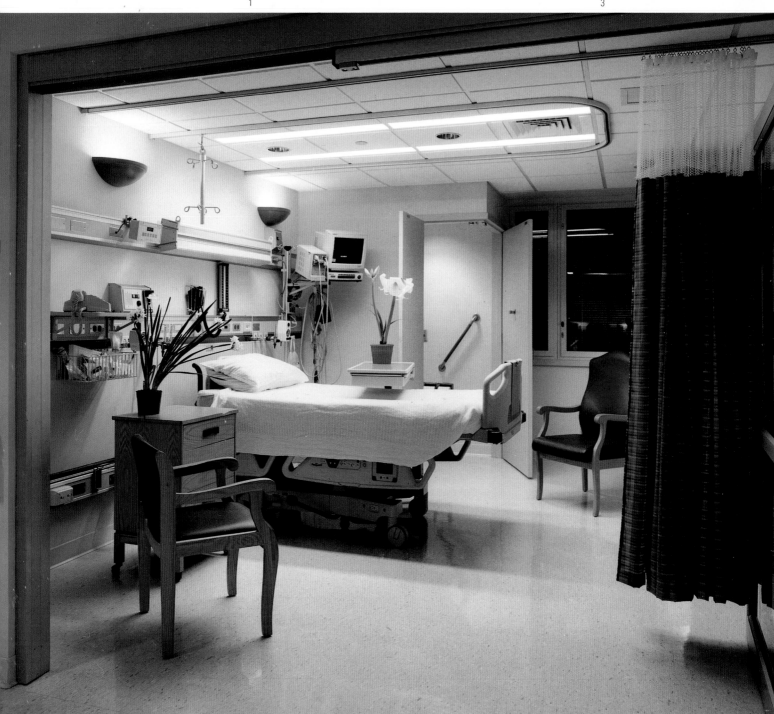

4

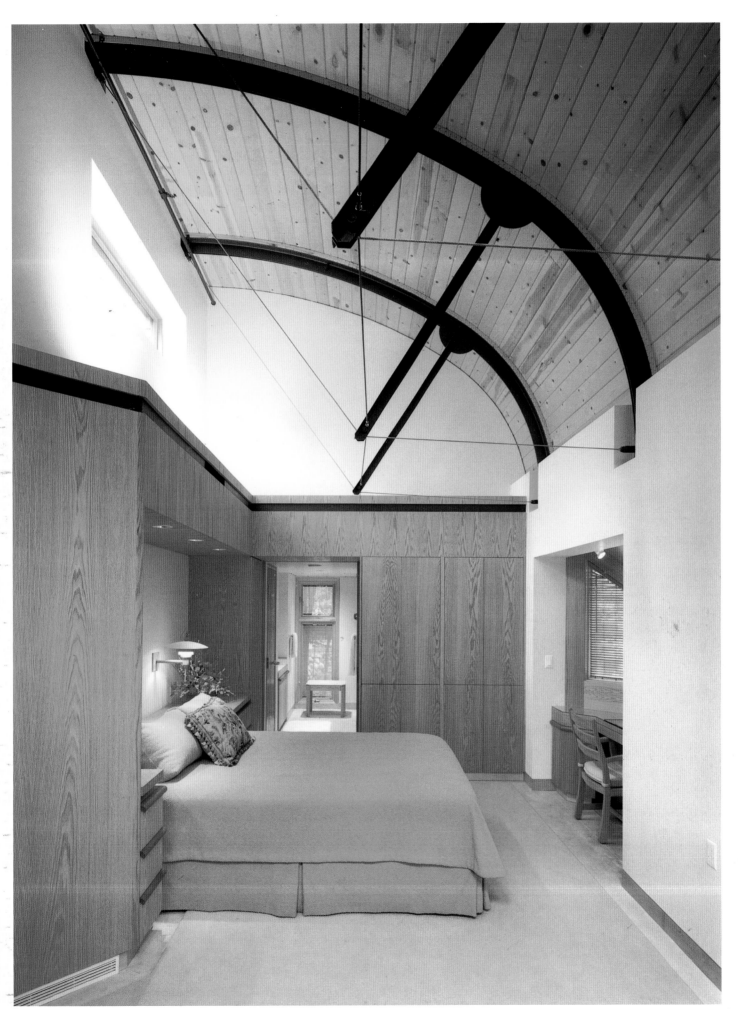

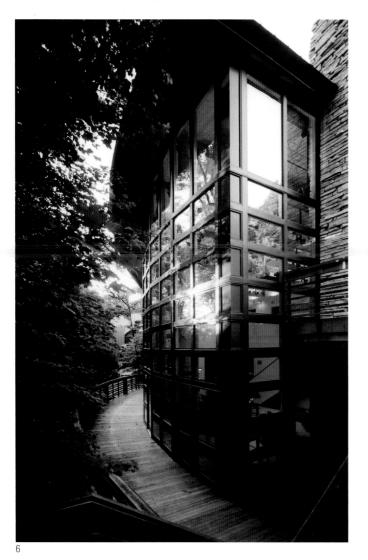

6

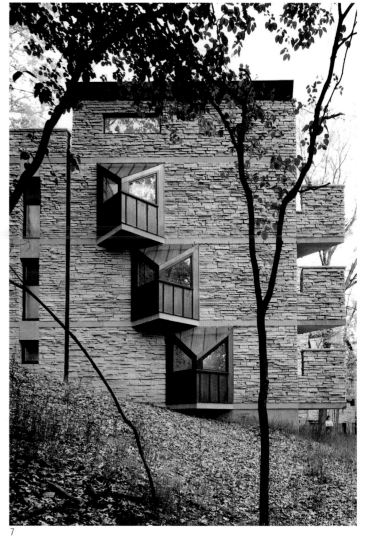

7

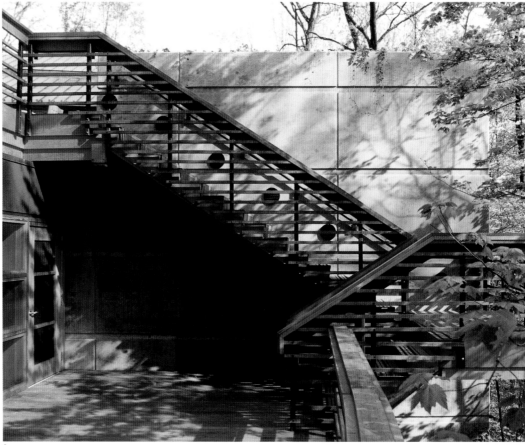

8

SEASONS: A Center for Renewal
Kalamazoo, Michigan, USA
HarleyEllis

6   Meeting House's exterior glass façade
7   Limestone clad north elevation
8   Exterior stairway connecting upper and
     lower decks
Opposite:
     Fireplace within meeting room
Following pages:
     Interior meeting room space
Photo credit: John Gilroy (6); Gay Quesada/
Hedrich-Blessing (7-10)

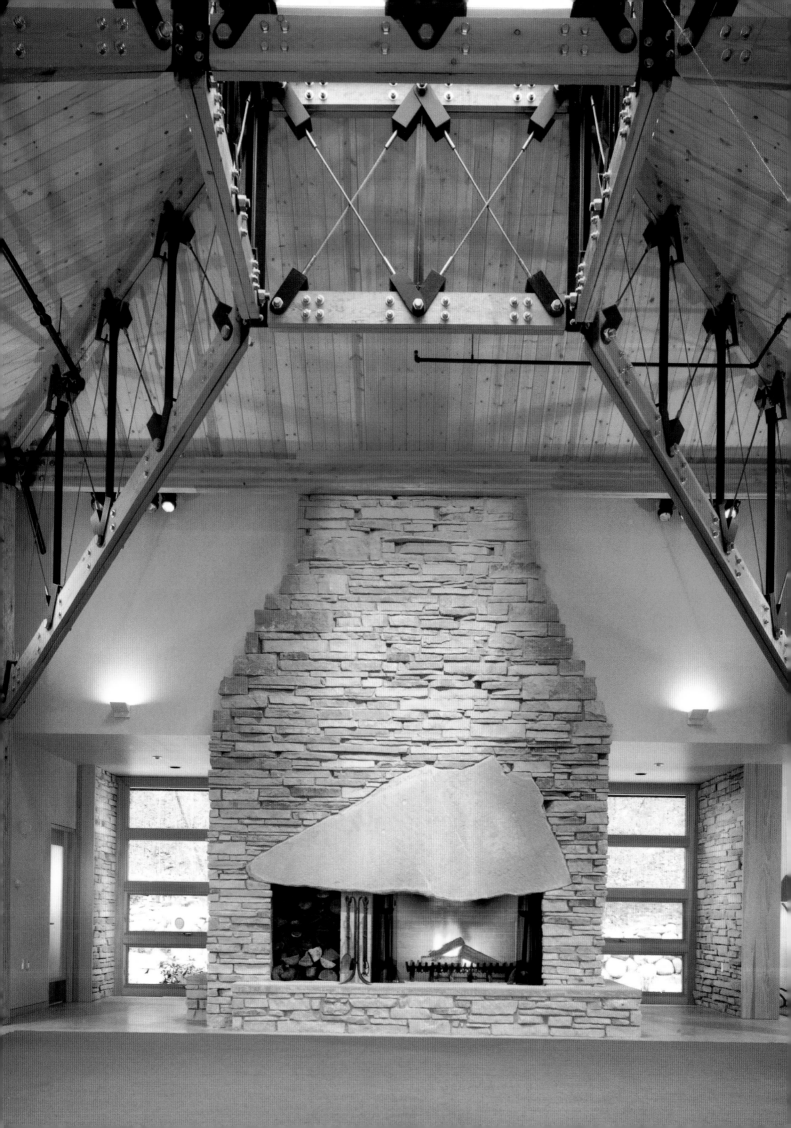

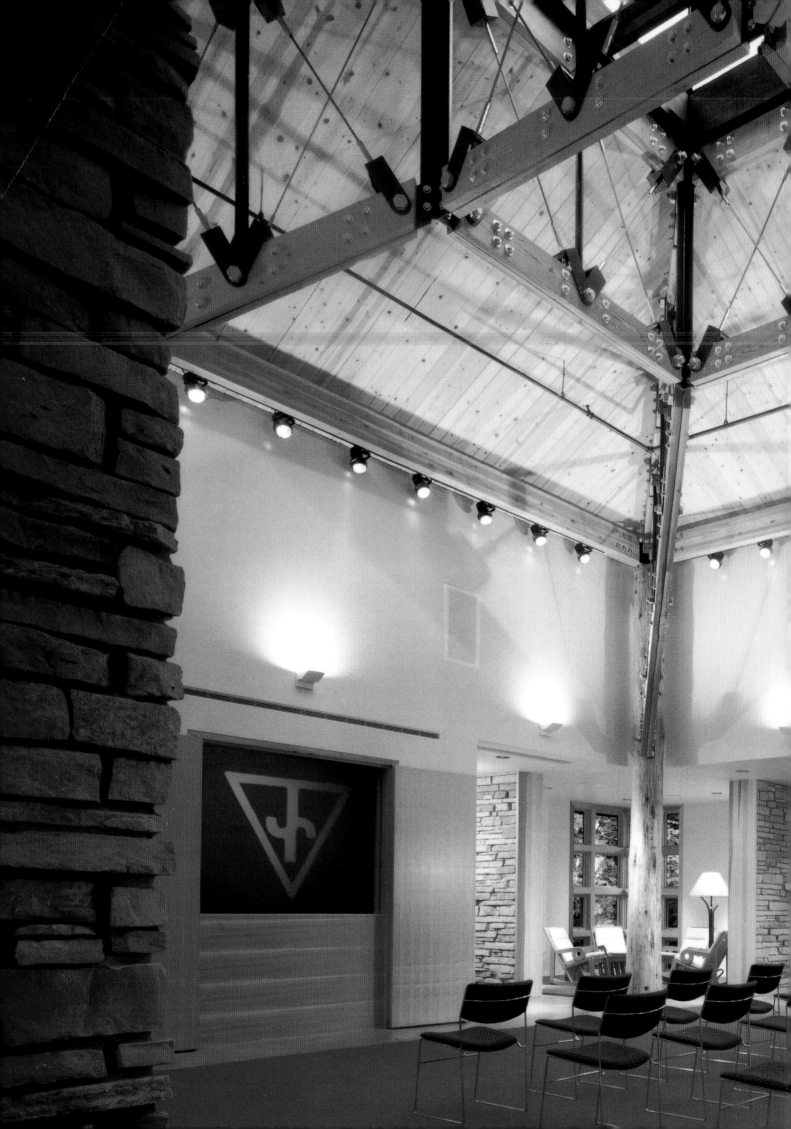

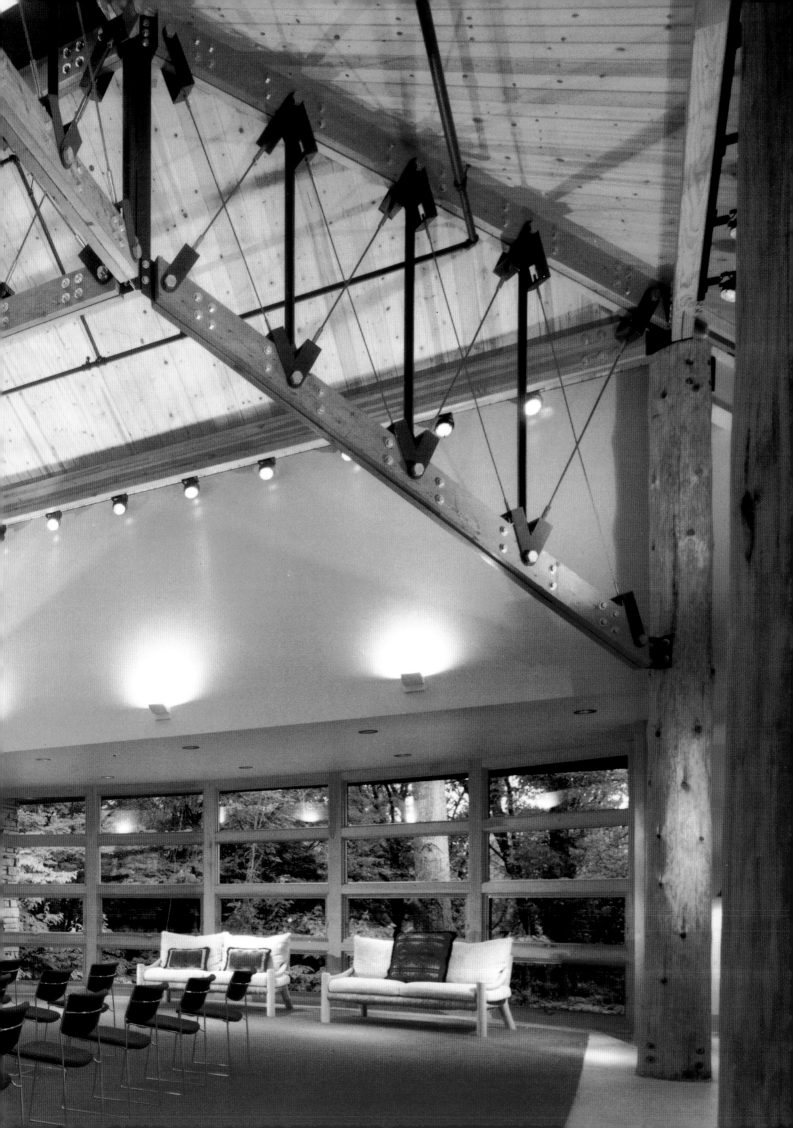

Biographies

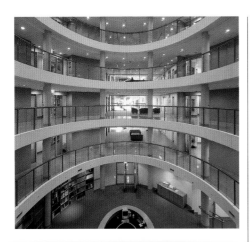

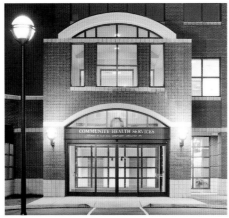

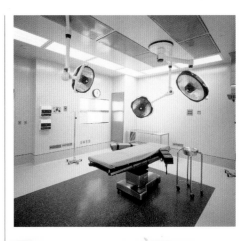

Ancher Mortlock and Woolley Architects

The practice was formed in 1946 when Sydney Ancher established his own firm. It became Ancher Mortlock and Murray in 1951 and gradually expanded until Ken Woolley left the Government Architect's Office of NSW to become a partner in 1964. Incorporation in 1969 allowed for smaller involvement shareholdings by young directors who have come and gone in furthering their careers.

Ken Woolley, current chairman and design director, is involved in the design output of the office to a greater or lesser degree, depending on the nature of the project. Ken has pursued a distinctive professional career though combining design talent with practical architectural knowledge. Other directors: Stephen Thomas, Dale Swan and Phil Baigent, and associates Lynn Vlismas, Garry Wallace and Robin Yeap work on particular projects in collaboration with Ken Woolley and other architects. Each member of the firm is selected for their commitment to excellence in design. Essentially this is a design studio approach and the practice is based on the concept of personal service to the client which has earned it many awards.

The practice has a strong commitment to involvement in the building vernacular of the day, not just by responding to it as a source of inspiration, but by taking part in its development and application. It works with pragmatic developer builders and market-oriented production design as much as with government clients and others concerned with architectural image and prestige.

Ancher Mortlock and Woolley Architects are proud to have also been responsible for the design of a number of significant venues for the Sydney 2000 Olympics.

Du Bose Associates, Inc. Architects

For four decades, Du Bose Associates, Inc. Architects has continuously built its award-winning practice, offering architectural, master planning, and interior design services, and providing thoughtful, and distinctive project solutions. The firm's emphasis is on superior quality, service, diversity, and identifying creative opportunities within each project.

In addition to Community Health Services, the Du Bose care portfolio includes a new entrance lobby; wayfinding and circulation enhancements; a geriatric care floor and a trauma center for Saint Francis Hospital and Medical Center; multiple projects for Veterans Benefits Administration; and Worchester Foundation for Experimental Biology.

Other aspects of the firm's architectural practice include:

- Planning, academic, residential, and library projects for a variety of prestigious colleges, universities, and independent schools.

- Headquarters, specialized facilities, and interior design for corporate insurance and financial service clients.

- Participation in the design of the new Hartford Public High School and the design of a new five-town sponsored Math Science and Technology Magnet Middle School.

- The Science Center of Connecticut soon to be constructed on the Connecticut River.

- Renovation enhancement and accessibility upgrades to more than 26 of Connecticut State Parks.

- Multiple projects for the US Postal Service.

Du Bose Associates, Inc. Architects' staff is made up of seasoned, dedicated professionals who are constantly studying and staying abreast of current techniques and technologies. The staff includes experts in the latest AutoCAD, graphic and 3D animation software packages.

The firm has offices in Hartford, Connecticut and Westerly, Rhode Island. The firm has been honoured with many awards such as: National AIA Award of Merit; Builder's Choice Awards; New England Health Care Design Awards; AIA Connecticut, Modern Office Technology; New York Construction News and the American Woodworking Institute; and 1999 International Masonry Institute New England Region Golden Trowel Awards.

HKS Inc.

HKS Inc. is in the forefront of designing healthcare facilities all over the world. It was founded in Dallas in 1939 and has additional offices in Orlando, Tampa, Los Angeles and Richmond. For six decades, HKS has provided planning, architectural and engineering services to a national and international clientele. In addition, it provides interior, structural, environmental graphics and construction administration services. The firm's portfolio of completed healthcare projects includes academic, ambulatory care, cancer, community, long-term, mental health, medical office buildings, research, children's and women's facilities.

HKS is consistently ranked as one of the top healthcare design firms in the nation—first in terms of value and volume of healthcare construction—according to *Modern Healthcare* magazine. We have been responsible for planning and designing over 450 healthcare projects representing more than 40,000 beds and 55 million square feet.

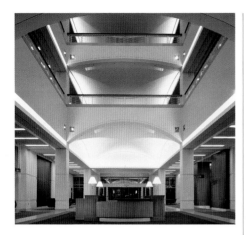

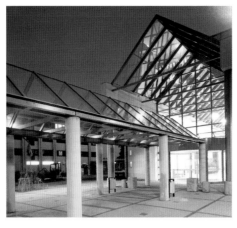

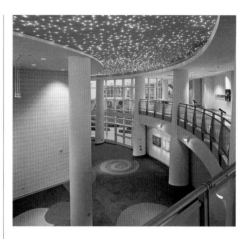

Hellmuth, Obata & Kassabaum, Inc.

Hellmuth, Obata & Kassabaum, Inc. (HOK) has specialized in the planning and design of healthcare facilities for more than 40 years. To date, HOK have completed projects worth over $2 billion in construction costs, including more than 400 separate projects in acute care, ambulatory care, long-term care facilities, senior housing, and medical office buildings.

HOK are working with progressive healthcare providers all over the world, literally redefining service delivery for the 21st Century. As a result, HOK know the important issues influencing the planning and design of healthcare facilities.

Properly planned and designed, the healthcare delivery setting of the 21st century will present a positive organizational image, promote a healing environment and enhance operational efficiencies. HOK is assisting clients in the development of new delivery models and facilities to meet the needs of the changing healthcare world. HOK partner with clients, becoming an intricate part of their vision and expressing that vision through the built environment.

Montois Partners

With the millennium, Montois Partners is celebrating 50 years of architecture.

Since its inception, the firm has brought to Belgium a sense of international style not seen before in the country on such a scale. Since the mid 1980s, to comply with a moving environment Montois Partners remains faithful to the modernistic vision and designs a more contextual architecture, with a revival to the modern movement today.

Projects such as the Hilton Brussels and the research centers of Texaco Europe and Solvay & Cie launched the firm as one of the largest in Belgium. The firm has designed many headquarters office buildings such as Citibank Belgium and Banque Indosuez, as well as embassies. It has experience in, virtually all, building types—newly built or renovated ones— including airports.

Montois Partners is probably the Belgian firm, which has the most experience in university and hospital design. The firm has designed hospitals in Africa and other European countries and is presently active in Eastern Europe and Turkey.

NBBJ

NBBJ is highly regarded as an international leader in architecture for healthcare. For nearly 60 years, on thousands of projects, it have redefined the role of architecture in promoting health, healing, influenced the relationship between contemporary medical practice and the patient, and set precedents that change the face of healthcare.

The firm's healthcare practice includes more than 300 specialists: architects and healthcare practitioners. Respected authorities in their fields of expertise, they lecture and publish regularly and participate actively in major international healthcare organizations and conferences.

NBBJ's work, which ranges from rural hospitals to urban medical centers, from birthing centers to high-tech treatment facilities, is informed by four guiding principles:

Knowledge

To have a profound understanding of healthcare: as an industry facing enormous pressure in an aggressive and competitive marketplace, burdened with complex rules and regulations; as institutions and systems struggling to keep pace with change; as a community of practitioners seeking to advance the science and art of healing.

Creativity

To seek clients who have a vision and who recognize the transformative architecture capacity. To continually challenge our clients and the firm to seek the unexpected and the exceptional, both in strategy and in its implementation.

Leadership

To lead clients through the decision making maze. By developing consensus among the diverse groups, each with its own valuable and distinct perspective, and by listening actively for insights and ideas on which to build and enlist all the participants in the authorship of the project.

Perspective

Perspective, experience studied and understood in context and translated into knowledge, is the key. It gives the firm the vision to unlock opportunities and solve problems. NBBJ use lessons learnt from all its work in retail, education, hospitality and other fields, to inform, inspire and add value to solutions for healthcare environments.

By setting the highest standard of design, for which accomplishments NBBJ has received numerous awards, and have demonstrated to the healthcare industry that the useful need not be utilitarian and that efficiency is no bar to excellence.

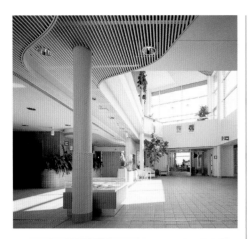

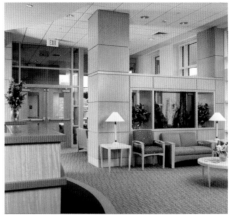

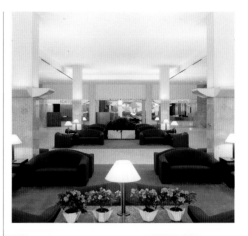

Paatela & Paatela, Architects Ltd.

The architectural practice of Paatela & Paatela, Architects was founded by Jussi and Toivo Paatela in 1919. The firm is now run by the third generation of Paatela architects. This makes it one of the oldest architectural firms in Finland.

In the course of its 80 years of operations, Paatela & Paatela has enhanced its expertise and experience, notably in the design of hospitals and other healthcare facilities and in the development of related functions. The firm has made a marked contribution to the construction of Finland's hospital network in the 1900s having been involved in the design and development of a number of university hospitals, central hospitals and health centres.

The new building for Turku University Central Hospital, one of the firm's most recent assignments, expresses the functional requirements, philosophy of care and construction solutions of a 'high-tech high-touch' hospital of the future, in a manner appropriate to the new millennium.

Due to the knowledge and experience gained by Paatela & Paatela, Architects in the healthcare sector, it has increasingly broadened its scope to include international projects. Among these are feasibility studies, preliminary sketch designs and full-scale architectural and functional design services for the construction of a whole range of facilities, from local health centres to major hospital complexes.

In addition to governmental, municipal and private clients, Paatela & Paatela, Architects has served as a consultant for Finnish construction companies, the Finnish International Development Agency, FINNIDA; Finland's Ministry for Foreign Affairs and various international healthcare organizations.

The most recent international projects undertaken by the firm are located in Russia and China. Finland's proximity to Russia and the Baltic countries gives the firm added value when offering healthcare design services to planners and investors in these countries. Paatela & Paatela, Architects also has design experience in a number of countries in Africa and the Middle East.

In addition to planning and design assignments, members of the practice have acted as consultants and lecturers for a range of prestigious clients including the Ministry of Public Health P.R. of China and the World Health Organisation (WHO).

TRO/The Ritchie Organization

TRO/The Ritchie Organization is a 180-person planning and design firm specialising in healthcare facilities. Services include architecture, planning, interior design and engineering. A closely-held C Corporation based in Newton, Massachusetts; the firm maintains regional offices in Birmingham, Alabama and Sarasota, Florida. TRO was established in 1909 and began building its healthcare expertise shortly thereafter. For the past 50 years, the firm has specialised exclusively in health-related facilities.

Currently, TRO is ranked among the top USA healthcare facilities design firms (*Modern Healthcare* Magazine, March 22 1999). TRO has completed a broad range of healthcare projects along the eastern seaboard and the Midwest. Its award-winning experience runs the gamut of healthcare facilities. Within its healthcare speciality, TRO's volume has encompassed over 400 clients with construction projects totalling more than four-and-a-half billion dollars.

Outstanding client service, coupled with a fundamental understanding of the ever-evolving demands of the healthcare delivery system, are at the forefront of TRO's business philosophy. Responsiveness, availability, commitment, constant communication and full team involvement are the cornerstones for the firm's success in project delivery.

TRO's architectural/engineering staff is trained in computer aided design and drafting (AutoCad 2000). The extensive network of workstations seamlessly integrates CADD programs with business applications to fully support the project. Project data and files are accessible throughout the office and e-mail is accessible to everyone, making it easy to share files with external members of the project team through e-mail attachments and FTP downloads. TRO also utilise the Internet to provide the most up-to-date research and information available.

The firm works with clients to define a standard of excellence that responds to their needs with flexibility, imagination and the highest quality design services. TRO's record of repeat business is over 90 percent. Client relationships have spanned decades, some for over 40 continuous years, attesting to clients' utmost satisfaction with our performance.

Woods Bagot

Woods Bagot is an international design and consulting firm that has been in continuous practice for 130 years. Founded in Adelaide, South Australia, the company is proud that its first client remains a client to this day. Operating from 11 offices in Australia, Asia and the Middle East, the company has over 350 staff with skills and experience extending across the full range of design services: architecture, planning, landscape design and interior design. It incorporates all aspects of consulting services, including but not limited to value management, needs analysis, strategic facility planning, design management and risk management.

Health planning and design has formed a core component of the Woods Bagot portfolio for 12 decades. In the past 10 years the practice has completed in excess of 200 hospital projects, over 90 of these in the last three years. Hospital projects in Australia and Asia range in value from less than $1 million to more than $200 million, indicating both the versatility of the practice and its ability to provide a consistent professional service, regardless of project size or complexity.

Woods Bagot has designed all types of health facilities, hospitals, medical centres, laboratories, even corporate fit-outs for hospital operators, and specialises in the upfront facility planning services that are the linchpin of a successful project.

Through a strategic alliance with Health Care of Australia, Woods Bagot has gained extensive experience in the private hospital sector, allowing the practice to become expert in cost-effective design solutions aimed at capital and recurrent cost reductions, commensurate with quality hospital environments. This has enabled Woods Bagot to attract an increasingly discerning clientele.

Woods Bagot has extensive and continuous experience in major public hospital work at tertiary teaching level and has developed high levels of knowledge and expertise relating to the most complex of clinical departments. Certain departments (eg. operating theatres) have been dealt with so many times that specialist health professionals in the company are dedicated solely to their design and delivery. These staff are expert in the state-of-the-art technology and philosophies relating to such specialist departments, ensuring an end project that satisfies the most demanding of users.

Index